OBSTETRIC AND GYNAECOLOGICAL
NURSING

NURSES' AIDS SERIES

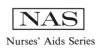

Nurses' Aids Series

OBSTETRIC AND GYNAECOLOGICAL NURSING

3rd Edition

Rosemary E. Bailey SRN, SCM, MTD, RNT, DN(Lond)
Director of Education, Royal Free Hospital, London;
Examiner to the General Nursing Council, Central Midwives Board and the
University of London;
Formerly Tutor in the Education Department, Royal College of Midwives,
Sister Tutor, St Bartholomew's Hospital, London

Jane Grayshon RGN, SCM, Dip.Life Sciences Nursing (Edin)
Formerly Research Sister, Department of Obstetrics and Gynaecology,
University of Nottingham,
Baillière Prizewinner for Nursing Studies, 1980

Baillière Tindall
London Philadelphia Toronto Sydney Tokyo

Baillière Tindall   24–28 Oval Road, London NW1 7DX
W. B. Saunders
The Curtis Center, Independence Square West
Philadelphia, PA 19106–3399, USA

55, Horner Avenue
Toronto, Ontario M8Z 4X6 Canada

Harcourt Brace Jovanovich (Australia) Pty Ltd.,
32–52 Smidmore Street, Marrickville, NSW 2204,
Australia

Harcourt Brace Jovanovich (Japan) Inc.,
Ichibancho Central Building, 22–1 Ichibancho,
Chiyoda-ku, Tokyo 102, Japan

© 1983 Baillière Tindall

First published 1969
Second edition 1975
Third edition 1983
  Reprinted 1985, 1987, 1989 and 1990

Printed in England by Clays Ltd, St Ives plc

British Library Cataloguing in Publication Data
Bailey, Rosemary E.
Obstetric and gynaecological nursing. — 3rd ed.
—(Nurses' aids series)
1. Gynaecologic nursing   2. Obstetrical nursing
I. Title   II. Grayshon, Jane R.   III. Series
610.73′678   RG951
ISBN 0-7020-0934-2

Contents

Preface

'Obstetric and Gynaecological Nursing' is a book for nurses which concentrates on the role of the nurse. The aim of this revision of Rosemary Bailey's informative book, is to help the nurse to consider and understand the special needs of the Obstetric or Gynaecological patient, and to direct her to channel her own expertise to meet those individual needs.

The nurse's role in Obstetrics and Gynaecology is outlined, with an emphasis on care and concern for the patient. In such a short book it is difficult both to convey factual information and to consider the impact of each condition on the patient: physiologically, psychologically, emotionally and socially. Occasionally I have sacrificed details of operative techniques to suggest the significance of procedures in the patient's life, in order that the reader can be attuned to the patient while she observes and learns the actual techniques in the ward situation. Where medical aspects are not covered, I hope that the reader will refer to other books as suggested in 'Further Reading'.

In areas which require special skill, such as in the Obstetric section where a midwife's expertise cannot be attained by a student nurse, I have suggested the role of the nurse within her limitations as a student. There is sufficient detail to prepare her to give first aid at a delivery.

I extend my thanks to my colleagues at the City Hospital, Nottingham, especially to Miss Anne Jequier, Dr Francoise Jadoule, and Mrs Dorothy Carter; to Miss Elaine Dove at Queen Margaret College, Edinburgh, and to Heather Reed for her contribution towards Chapter 14. I must also thank the many patients, especially Jenny Williams who has taught me so much by her honest discussions about what is helpful or unhelpful in nursing and midwifery. Also thanks are extended to Mr Geoffrey Gilbert for the photographs. Finally my thanks go to Rosemary Long for her guidance, and to my husband Matthew for his warm encouragement throughout every stage of my writing.

Jane Grayshon
August 1982

We gratefully acknowledge permission to reproduce the following: Fig. 7.9(c), Crowdys Wood Products Ltd; Fig. 24.2, Professor Sir John Dewhurst.

1 Patients and Nurses in Obstetrics and Gynaecology

Obstetric and gynaecological nursing is quite different from any other nursing, and calls for specialist skills in order to identify and meet the patient's needs. This chapter discusses the distinctive features of obstetric and gynaecological nursing, and the patient's individual needs are dealt with in detail with each condition.

Embarrassment One of the outstanding features of obstetrics and gynaecology is its very intimate nature. Every patient is expected to remove her clothes to be examined. She becomes very vulnerable because her 'private parts' are exposed.

The embarrassment and fear which the patient experiences are helped by the nurse's understanding and sympathy. One of the most important things a nurse can do is to remain sensitive to each patient. A female nurse is in an advantaged position to do this, because with a little imagination she can identify the patient's feelings and take action accordingly.

Emotional involvement Secondly, obstetrics and gynaecology is different because it demonstrates clearly the interaction between the physical and emotional aspects of life. The nurse has to care for a complete person, not parts of a person, because interrelated parts cannot be separated.

Obstetrics and gynaecology involves women only, and therefore women's reactions and emotions are prominent. Most women are aware that their moods change at different times during the month, as hormonal patterns change. The nurse in obstetrics and gynaecology often sees great alterations in the patient's mood, associated with menstruation (see Chapter 2), pregnancy (Chapter 4), the puerperium (Chapter 9) and at the menopause (Chapter 17).

The obstetric patient The obstetric patient, unlike other patients, is normally fit and well. She is taking part in one of the most natural and essential events in the history of mankind. She is thus not grateful for being made better, in the same way that patients are in other areas of medicine. She has been *persuaded* to attend for care and the nurse in obstetrics is, in one sense, on trial. If clinics or hospitals are uninviting or unfriendly, the patient is less likely to return, and the staff inevitably fail to reach their goal which is to promote health, detect abnormality and prevent complications. This could be an important contributing factor to Britain's relatively slow fall in the perinatal mortality rates (see Chapter 14). Each nurse individually plays a part in creating the atmosphere in clinics, and each one should, with other health care workers, endeavour to improve the standards and acceptability of obstetric care.

Secondly, the obstetric patient is different because she takes an active part in making decisions about the management of pregnancy, labour and the care of her baby. In other areas of medicine, the patient is often more passive whilst being cured; but the obstetric patient needs explanations, for example about the nature of antenatal tests, because she contributes her own opinions before a midwife or doctor can intervene. Patients and hospital staff thus actively work together, in order to do their best for a third party, the baby.

Thirdly, home and family are not peripheral considerations,

but they are central to the obstetric patient. The nurse has the opportunity to visualize the patient's place in her family and in the community, and to work towards the integration of the new baby to home and community life.

Fourthly, the obstetric patient is particularly receptive to health education and parentcraft instruction, and the nurse can learn how to teach patients about health care.

The gynaecological patient Gynaecological nursing demands skills as in any surgical ward, but calls for special sensitivity in order to meet the individual needs of the patient. Whereas some other disorders or operations can be laughed off or treated lightly, gynaecological conditions cannot be in the same way, because they threaten deep natural instincts. The very nature of gynaecology highlights the patient's part in reproduction and in the continuance of the human race.

Gynaecological nursing deals with two very important aspects of being a woman: *feminity* and *fertility*. It involves the core or the female's anatomy, that which distinguishes her from the male. Gynaecological surgery thus affects a patient's own body image: she not only loses a part of herself, but a part which is important to her very concept of herself as a woman. Similarly, hormone changes involve those hormones which give female characteristics and these also affect fertility.

Sexual relationships are often affected by gynaecological disorders and many women fear that an operation may change their husbands' feelings for them. The nurse must remember that sexual relationships play an important part in a happy marriage.

Embarrassment about the personal nature of gynaecology inhibits some patients from sharing with anyone but the nurse about their condition. This puts the nurse in the unique position of being the *only* person to whom the patient can turn for help or understanding. The nurse therefore has an important role in treating this information confidentially.

For all these reasons the patient may be tense and emotional, and seemingly unimportant happenings can lead to tears. To deal with these situations the nurse has not only to understand the patient, but to convey that understanding to her. Intelligence and imagination are required, to see the reasons behind the defensive attitude, perhaps the overt anxiety to please, or the feeling of isolation and embarrassment displayed by the patient, her husband, fiancé or other relatives. If these individual and human needs should pass unobserved, the key to gynaecological nursing will be lost from the very beginning.

2 The Menstrual Cycle

THE OVARY

The ovaries are two glandular structures lying on the posterior surface of the broad ligament below the uterine tube (Fig. 2.1). They develop in the germinal ridges on the posterior abdominal wall and during fetal life descend into the pelvis in the same manner as the testes. They are dull

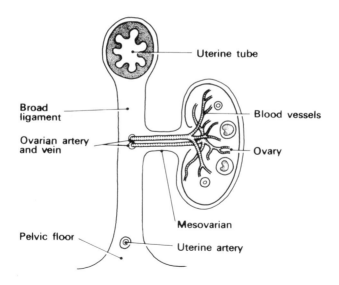

Fig. 2.1 Lateral view of the broad ligament showing the ovary outside the peritoneal cavity.

white in colour and corrugated on the surface, measuring 3 cm in length, 2 cm in width and 1 cm in thickness. Their weight is between 5 and 8 g.

Structure

The ovary consists of a medulla and cortex surrounded by a layer of germinal epithelium. The medulla is the central core and is continuous with the connective tissue of the broad ligament at the hilum where the blood vessels and lymphatics enter. The cortex contains the primary oocytes embedded in connective tissue. The germinal epithelium is a modified form of peritoneum which covers the ovary. Its blood supply is from the ovarian artery, a branch of the aorta, and the venous drainage is to the ovarian veins; the lymphatics drain to glands on the posterior abdominal wall and the nerve supply reaches the ovary from the pelvic plexus.

Function

The function of the ovary is twofold: to prepare the body for conception and gestation; and to deal with the period of gestation itself.

This second function will be enlarged upon in Chapter 4, 'Physiology and Management of Pregnancy'.

At birth the female is richly endowed with primary oocytes which in time will mature and become ova, although for the first 10 to 11 years of life they lie dormant. At puberty changes take place because of the action of the pituitary hormones and the so-called secondary sex characteristics develop: the breasts enlarge, the hips broaden and menstruation occurs for the first time. This is the *menarche*. At the same time these hormones have psychological effects such as are described in Chapter 1 and on page 10.

The ovaries contain some 200 000 primordial follicles, about 400 of which will eventually mature. Whilst the fetus is still in utero, maturation begins and many more layers of cells surround the ovum. This is followed by the appearance of fluid between the layers, the liquor folliculi. These cystic follicles are known as graafian follicles, which remain quite small until puberty is reached.

The action of the anterior pituitary hormones causes a cycle to commence, known as the menstrual cycle.

THE MENSTRUAL CYCLE

The menstrual cycle is a straightforward series of events in which various changes occur in order to prepare for a pregnancy. Whenever pregnancy does not occur, the cycle recommences, normally every 28 or 30 days, but sometimes every 21 to 42 days.

There are three main organs involved with the menstrual cycle: the pituitary gland, the ovary, and the uterus. Each of these organs has its own 'cycle', closely interlinked and dependent upon the others (Fig. 2.2).

The pituitary cycle

The production of follicle-stimulating hormone from the anterior pituitary gland, which stimulates the graafian follicle to ripen, increases until ovulation when it gradually declines. At ovulation, the pituitary produces the luteinizing hormone which stimulates the production of the corpus luteum.

The pituitary gland itself is under the influence of the hypothalamus which produces releasing factors until suppressed by feedback mechanisms.

The ovarian cycle

Following stimulation, one graafian follicle rapidly increases in size and protrudes from the surface of the ovary (Fig. 2.3). Tension increases and the ovarian covering stretches, thins and finally ruptures, often accompanied by a little pelvic pain (Mittelschmerz). Ovulation takes place each month from alternate ovaries, that is, each ovary ovulates at two-monthly intervals. It is possible for more than one ovum to be discharged at a time, especially after a period of suppression, and this results in dissimilar multiple pregnancies.

Once the ovum is shed, the empty follicle collapses and a

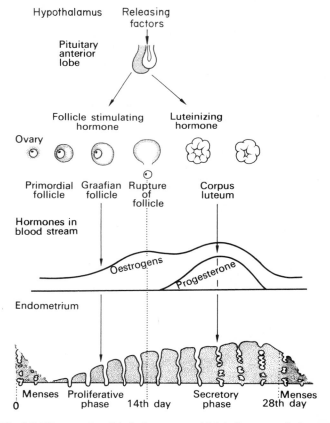

Fig. 2.2 Diagram showing the hormones which influence ovulation and the menstrual cycle.

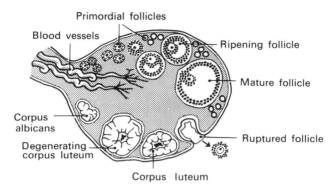

Fig. 2.3 Diagram to show the sequence of changes occurring in the ovum during each menstrual cycle.

little bleeding occurs into the cavity. The remaining membrana granulosa cells proliferate under the influence of the luteinizing hormone, and in a few days form a solid grey-coloured mass, the corpus luteum. The corpus luteum continues to grow for 14 days, after which it degenerates if fertilization has not occurred, and in nine months' time the only evidence is a small scar on the ovary. This cycle continues from puberty to the menopause and is only interrupted in a healthy woman by pregnancy.

The ovaries in their turn produce hormones. The granulosa cells of the graafian follicle produce a group of hormones known as oestrogens which are stored in the liquor folliculi from whence they pass into the systemic circulation. The corpus luteum continues the production of oestrogens and in addition produces progesterone.

The uterine cycle

Accompanying the pituitary and ovarian cycles is a series of endometrial changes. When menstruation occurs the endo-metrium is shed down to its basal layer, then under the influence of oestrogens it regenerates and thickens. This is the proliferative phase and lasts about ten days. Following ovulation and the production of progesterone the endometrium becomes even thicker, the glands more tortuous and full of secretions and the blood supply is enriched. This is the secretory phase and lasts 14 days, after which the lining is shed once more. The menstrual phase occurs 14 days after ovulation if fertilization has not taken place. The endometrium above the basal layer degenerates, due to spasm in the arteries and deprivation of blood flow, necrosis occurs and the lining sloughs off to be expelled from the uterus by muscular contraction. The menstrual flow continues for about five days and the blood loss is some 50 to 100 ml.

The general effects of ovarian hormones

The *oestrogens* bring about the changes which occur at puberty: the development of the breasts, widening of the hips, deposition of fat over the shoulders, and distribution of the axillary and pubic hair. (The growth of hair is stimulated by testosterone.) During the menstrual cycle, oestrogens govern the proliferative phase of the endometrium, stimulating growth and vascularization. They increase cervical secretion, producing a favourable medium for spermatozoa. During pregnancy the very high levels suppress ovulation, stimulate the growth of uterine muscle and the duct system of the breasts, and inhibit lactation until delivery. They help to retain calcium in bones, hence after the menopause many women develop osteoporosis.

Progesterone governs the secretory phase of the uterine cycle, increasing endometrial gland secretion. It stimulates growth of breast gland alveoli, causing premenstrual fullness and tingling. In pregnancy it influences the growth of the uterine decidua, relaxes smooth muscle, stimulates the growth of the alveoli in the breasts and together with oestrogens causes the retention of water and electrolytes that can be seen in the menstrual cycle and pregnancy.

The hygiene of menstruation

Many women experience a certain amount of discomfort just before and during menstruation. Much of this is due to the alteration in circulating hormones, but a few symptoms such as fullness in the pelvis and vague pain in the back are probably due to pelvic congestion. These discomforts can be alleviated by a hot bath and a mild analgesic, and plenty of exercise to improve circulation.

Added attention to hygiene is necessary at this time. Women must remember to wash frequently, to wear clean underwear each day and to change pads or tampons at least three times per day. Internal tampons are convenient and prevent unpleasant odour, and they can be used by all except the very young who in some cases should consult a doctor first in case the hymen is tight and insertion would cause pain. Few obstetricians raise objections to the use of tampons providing care is taken that the last tampon used has been removed, otherwise this could lead to infection and vaginal discharge.

Vaginal deodorants can alter the normal flora, and give rise to dermatitis around the vulva. Their use should not be necessary if women take adequate care to maintain hygiene.

The nurse must be ready to dispel many of the old wives' tales surrounding this subject. No harm will come from taking a bath or washing the hair during menstruation.

3 Physiology of Reproduction

THE UTERUS

The uterus is a hollow pear-shaped organ situated in the pelvic cavity, about 7.5 cm long, 5 cm wide and 2.5 cm deep, weighing about 60 g (Fig. 3.1).

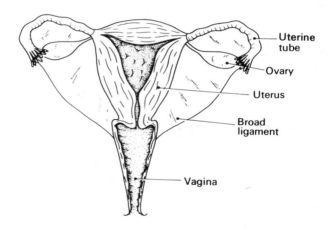

Fig. 3.1 The uterus and its appendages.

It consists of the corpus, the cervix and the isthmus (Fig 3.2).

The *corpus*, or body, comprises the upper two-thirds and encloses a triangular cavity. The uterine tubes enter the body at the cornua and the part above this is called the fundus.

The *cervix*, or neck, is cylindrical in shape and communicates with the cavity above by the internal os and with the vagina below by the external os. The lower half projects into the vault of the vagina.

The *isthmus* is the area joining cervix to corpus, it assumes great importance in pregnancy.

Structure

The uterus is composed of plain muscle which is arranged in a spiral form running from the cornua to the cervix, giving a circular effect along the uterine tube and cervix, and an oblique effect over the corpus (Fig. 3.3). This muscle is called the myometrium and its main function is to expel the fetus from the birth canal during labour.

The lining is endometrium, which in the reproductive years is constantly changing (Chapter 2). The perimetrium is a double fold of peritoneum which is reflected from the top of

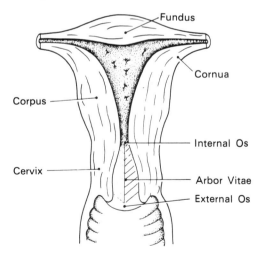

Fig. 3.2 Divisions of the uterus.

the bladder at the level of the internal os, envelops the uterus and uterine tubes, then posteriorly at the level of the external os makes a deep pocket known as the pouch of Douglas before covering the rectum (Fig. 3.4).

The muscle of the cervix is continuous with that of the corpus. The upper two-thirds of the canal is lined by columnar epithelium containing deep, tubular glands, and the lower third by stratified squamous epithelium continuous

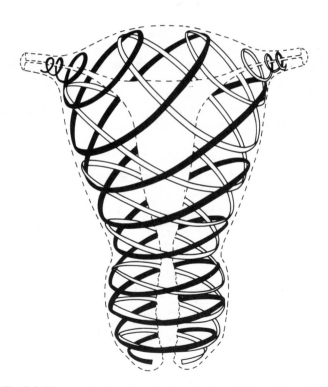

Fig. 3.3 Diagram to show the spiral arrangement of the uterine muscle fibres.

with the lining of the vagina and covering of the cervix. This squamocolumnar junction is of importance as it is here that carcinoma often occurs (Chapter 24).

The uterus has a rich blood supply from the uterine and ovarian arteries which anastomose freely (Fig. 3.5). Venous drainage is by veins of the same name, lymphatic drainage is to the lumbar and hypogastric nodes, and the nerve supply is sympathetic and parasympathetic.

The supports of the uterus

The supports of the uterus are described in detail in Chapter 26. The muscles of the pelvic floor (see Figs. 26.1 and 26.2) help the uterus to remain in position, with the transverse cervical ligaments, uterosacral ligaments, and pubocervical ligaments (see Fig. 26.3). The round ligaments assist in keeping the uterus in its normal anteverted (forward tilted), anteflexed (bent on itself) position (Fig. 3.6).

Excessive strain on the uterine supports during pregnancy

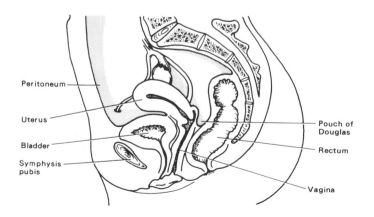

Fig. 3.4 Sagittal section of the pelvic organs.

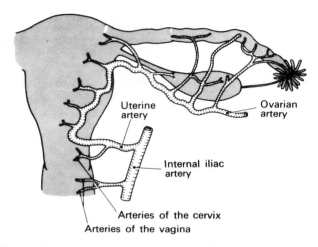

Uterine artery

Ovarian artery

Internal iliac artery

Arteries of the cervix

Arteries of the vagina

Fig. 3.5 The blood supply to the uterus and its appendages.

or labour predisposes to genital prolapse later in life.

Note. The broad ligaments are folds of peritoneum continuous with the covering of the uterus and extending to the side wall of the pelvis. Despite their name they are not ligaments, and in no way support the uterus.

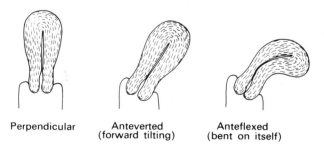

Perpendicular

Anteverted (forward tilting)

Anteflexed (bent on itself)

Fig. 3.6 Diagram to show how the normal position of the uterus is achieved (sagittal section).

DEVELOPMENT AND EMBEDDING OF THE OVUM

The development of the ovum and the sequence of events when fertilization does not occur are described in Chapter 2. If the ovum is fertilized, the sequence of events changes.

Maturation
Prior to ovulation certain changes have taken place within the graafian follicle known as maturation, whereby the ovum is able to reduce the chromosomes in the nucleus from 46 to 23, the remainder being extruded as a polar body (Fig. 3.7).

Fertilization
After ovulation the ovum is caught up in the uterine tube and is wafted slowly towards the uterus (see Chapter 27). Fertilization usually occurs in the tube, where the strongest of some 300 million spermatozoa have swum from the vagina after intercourse. Abnormal spermatozoa tend not to survive this rather rigorous journey, thus nature tries to safeguard the next generation.

Every normal human cell carries 46 chromosomes: 22 pairs of autosomes and 1 pair of sex chromosomes. The ovum, with its 23 chromosomes after maturation, is penetrated by a single spermatozoon, which also carries 23 chromosomes. Thus, half the mother's chromosomes unite with half the father's, to form a whole cell with 46 chromosomes. This single fertilized cell will continue to grow and divide, and becomes a whole human being.

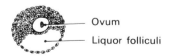

Ovum
Liquor folliculi

Fig. 3.7 Graafian follicle.

When the two sex chromosomes halve, the mother's (XX) can only be an X, but the father's (XY) can be either X or Y: thus it is the male who determines the sex of the fetus.

Growth

The fertilized cell grows quickly by cell division, the initial cell dividing into two, two into four and so on (Fig. 3.8).

This small ball of cells somewhat resembles a mulberry, and is called a *morula*. Cell differentiation occurs very early;

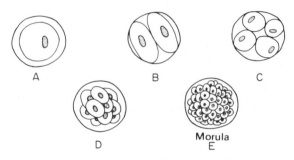

Fig. 3.8 Diagram of the fertilized ovum undergoing cell division.

this is an important fact because serious consequences may follow damage such as by drugs, irradiation, or maternal infection. The destruction of one cell could mean the absence of an organ or limb.

Once the morula has formed, a small cystic space begins to appear, pushing the bulk of the cells to one end. The outer layer is known as the *trophoblast* and the mass of cells the *inner cell mass*. The whole is called the *blastocyst* (Fig. 3.9).

It is at this stage that the fertilized ovum enters the uterine cavity, four days after fertilization, five to six days after ovulation. The trophoblast develops quickly and is concerned with absorbing nutrition and secreting a hormone—chorionic

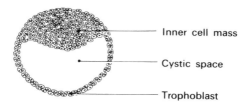

Fig. 3.9 Blastocyst.

gonadotrophin. At this stage it is ready to embed in the endometrium.

The activity of hormones in relation to this growth is represented in Fig. 3.10.

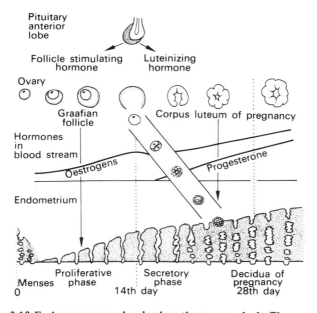

Fig. 3.10 Early pregnancy, showing how the ovum embeds. The corpus luteum persists and menstruation does not occur.

Embedding

When the blastocyst reaches the uterine lining it secretes a ferment which digests the endometrial cells and causes a small depression in which the blastocyst lies. As digestion continues, it sinks further into the thickened endometrium, now termed the decidua, until finally it is buried in the decidua and the site of entry sealed with a fibrin plug (Fig. 3.11).

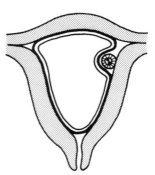

Fig. 3.11 Implantation of the ovum in the upper segment of the uterus.

Trophoblast

The trophoblastic cells multiply and differentiate into three layers.

1. The *syncitiotrophoblast* or *syncitium*—the outer layer, where the protoplasm is not enclosed by cell walls.

2. *Cytotrophoblast* or *Langhans' layer*, well-differentiated cells.

3. *Loose connective tissue* into which blood vessels grow.

Over the trophoblast small projections or villi appear, similar to the intestinal villus and composed of the layers mentioned above, but these develop still further, branching like a tree, and are known as chorionic villi (Fig. 3.12).

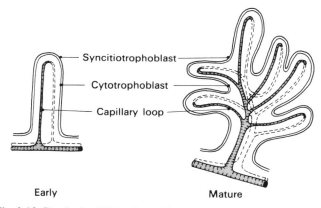

Fig. 3.12 Chorionic villi (early and late).

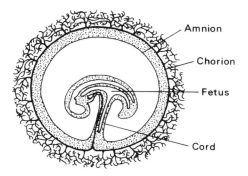

Fig. 3.13 Development of the true chorionic villi and the fetus in the liquor amnii.

Chorionic villi surround the whole embryo, some are favourably situated with regard to the blood sinuses, these grow rapidly and obtain nutrition for the growing embryo. Others eventually degenerate leaving a thin membrane in their place. At about 12 weeks the process is complete and the circular plaque of villi is known as the placenta, whilst the degenerated membranous area is the chorion (Fig. 3.13).

Development of the fetus

Whilst the above processes have been going on, the inner cell mass also undergoes development. The stage of *gestation* is estimated according to the number of weeks after the last menstrual period. However, as fertilization normally occurs two weeks after that day (on day 14 of the cycle), the age of the *fetus* is actually two weeks behind the gestational date.

The pregnancy test is usually positive when a woman is two weeks late with her expected period, so her pregnancy is calculated as six weeks gestation. The gestation period of a normal pregnancy is 40 weeks.

Details of stages of development of the fetus are given in weeks of gestation below.

4 weeks	Head, tail fold and limb buds. Length 1 cm.
6 weeks	Heart beats (seen on ultrasound scan).
12 weeks	Fingers and toes are formed and nails are forming. Length 9 cm. Passes small amounts of urine.
16 weeks	Movements begin (felt at 17–20 weeks).
20 weeks	Hair and lanugo (down hair on the skin) appear. Length 25 cm.
28 weeks	Eyelids separated, skin red, head large in proportion to the body. Length 35 cm. Weight 1250 g.
36 weeks	Pink in colour, covered with vernix caseosa, a sebaceous substance which protects the skin. Length 45 cm. Weight 2500 g.
40 weeks	Length 50 cm. Weight 3500 g.

THE FETUS AND PLACENTA AT TERM

The fetus

The fetus at term is about 50 cm in length and weighs about 3500 g, it is pale pink in colour and has laid down subcutaneous fat. There may be some lanugo present and the hair on the scalp is some 2 to 3 cm in length. The skin is smooth, and covered with a sebaceous secretion known as vernix caseosa. The nails reach the ends of the fingers and toes.

The internal organs are developed to a stage where the fetus can exist independently, although some are not fully mature. The bowel is filled with meconium, a greenish-black substance, rather sticky and composed of bile pigments, alimentary secretions, desquamated cells, lanugo and liquor amnii which have been swallowed.

The head is still large in comparison with the body, and its anatomy is important as this is the largest and hardest part to pass through the birth canal.

The fetal skull The skull is composed of the face, the base and the vault. The face and base are ossified at birth, but the bones of the vault are not. The vault consists of two *frontal* bones, two *temporal* bones, two *parietal* bones and one *occipital* bone. These are flat bones which have been laid down in membrane, ossification commencing about the seventh week of gestation, near their centre and slowly radiating outwards. At birth, membranous areas can be felt on the skull, those lying between the bones being called sutures, and where the sutures meet, fontanelles (Fig. 3.14).

The anterior fontanelle, or bregma, is the meeting place of four sutures, and is diamond shaped. The posterior fontanelle, or lambda, is triangular in shape where three sutures meet, and is smaller than the bregma.

The sutures and fontanelles are important in labour as they allow alteration in the diameters of the skull, known as moulding. By pressure on one diameter, the bones override each other and the diameter is decreased, the one at right angles being correspondingly increased to accommodate the contents of the skull. The sutures and fontanelles are also

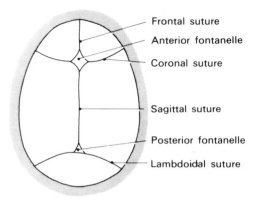

Fig. 3.14 The fetal skull showing sutures and fontanelles.

important in diagnosis, in labour they help to confirm the position and presentation of the fetus as they can be felt by the examining finger during vaginal examination. After birth the width of the suture helps confirm the maturity or otherwise of the baby.

The bregma does not ossify completely until 18 months after birth, but the lambda closes soon after birth. The mother may need reassurance that these areas cannot be damaged easily.

The diameters of the skull (Fig. 3.15) are of significance during labour because descent of the head is easiest when the smallest diameters pass through the birth canal. The diameter which comes down first depends on which region of the fetal skull comes first (called the presenting part); this in turn depends on the amount of flexion of the fetal head. When the head is well flexed down on to the chest, the vertex is presenting and the engaging diameter is the suboccipito-bregmatic diameter of 9.5 cm.

During the antenatal period, the biparietal diameter is of significance because this grows at a predictable rate and its

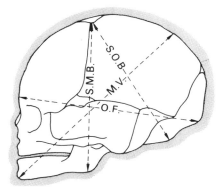

Fig. 3.15 **Lateral view of the fetal skull showing some of the diameters.**
S.O.B.; suboccipito-bregmatic, 9.5 cm. O.F.; occipito-frontal,
11.4 cm. M.V.; mento-vertical, 13.3 cm. S.M.B.; submento-
bregmatic, 9.5 cm.

measurement using ultrasound scan can not only confirm
fetal maturity, but also serial scans can check that growth is
continuing normally.

The fetal circulation The fetal blood is quite separate from
the mother's blood. Oxygen and nutrients pass by diffusion
from the mother's blood, and likewise carbon dioxide and
waste products diffuse from the fetal blood to be excreted by
the mother.

The fetal circulation differs from that of the adult because
the blood is oxygenated in the placenta and not in the lungs. It
is a much less efficient method and therefore there are several
added requirements.

1. A higher haemoglobin content in order to pick up the
maximum amount of oxygen.
2. A modified form of haemoglobin (HbF) which is active
in a slightly more acid blood.

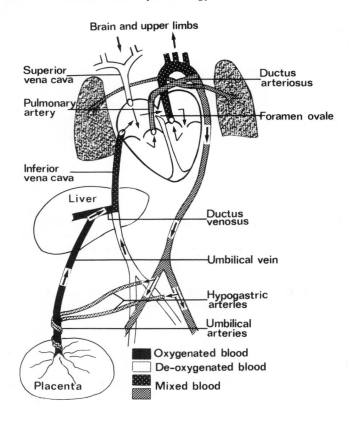

Fig. 3.16 Fetal circulation.

3. Certain anatomical structures: (*a*) the ductus venosus; (*b*) the ductus arteriosus; (*c*) the foramen ovale; (*d*) the two hypogastric arteries (Fig. 3.16).

The route of the blood All veins travel to the heart, and arteries travel from it, and the fetal circulation is no different.

The umbilical vein carries oxygenated blood to the fetus, and two umbilical arteries carry deoxygenated blood from the fetus to the placenta.

Oxygen diffuses from the maternal blood in the chorio-decidual space to the placental villi, the vessels of which unite to form the umbilical vein which travels along the cord to the fetus. After passing through the abdominal wall at the umbilicus, the main vessel, known as the *ductus venosus*, joins the inferior vena cava while a branch carries blood straight to the liver. The oxygenated blood now mixes with a little deoxygenated blood coming up from the lower trunk and legs in the inferior vena cava as it is carried to the heart. There the blood is directed across from the right atrium to the left atrium, through the *foramen ovale*. After passing from the left atrium to the left ventricle, the blood leaves the heart via the aorta and supplies oxygenated blood to the vital centres in the brain and the rest of the body. Blood from the head and neck, returning through the superior vena cava to the right atrium, is directed across the flow coming from the inferior vena cava to enter the right ventricle which it leaves by the pulmonary artery.

A small stream passes through the pulmonary artery to the lungs but the majority of the blood by-passes the lungs through a large vessel, the *ductus arteriosus*, which connects the pulmonary artery to the aorta beyond the branches leading to the head, neck and shoulders. The deoxygenated blood leaves the common iliac arteries by the *hypogastric arteries*, which pass outwards to the umbilicus and enter the cord as the umbilical arteries. Blood travels back to the placenta where reoxygenation takes place.

The placenta

The placenta at term is about 20 cm in diameter and about one-sixth of the weight of the fetus, or 600 g. It has two surfaces: the maternal and fetal surfaces.

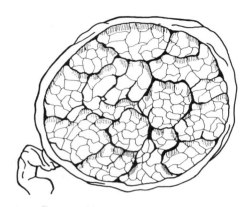

Fig. 3.17 The placenta: maternal surface showing cotyledons.

The maternal surface (Fig. 3.17). The maternal surface is attached to the uterine decidua and is deep red in colour. It is divided by deep grooves, or sulcii, into about 20 lobes known as cotyledons. This surface is made up of masses of villi.

The fetal surface (Fig. 3.18). The fetal surface lies adjacent to the fetus and is covered by amnion which can be stripped off to the point at which the cord is inserted. The vessels can be seen radiating out from the cord towards the periphery where they disappear from sight.

The chorion The chorion is an opaque membrane, continuous with the edge of the maternal surface of the placenta and lining the uterine cavity.

The amnion The amnion is the inner membrane, tough and shiny, and is continuous with the outer covering of the cord. Its cells secrete the liquor amnii which fills the amniotic cavity during pregnancy, and at term measures about a litre.

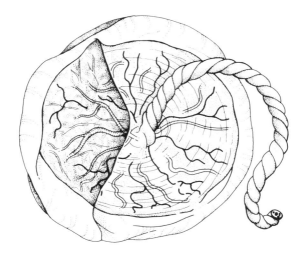

Fig. 3.18 The placenta: fetal surface with umbilical cord.

The cord The cord is about 50 cm in length and 2 cm in thickness. It is composed of a jelly-like material known as Wharton's jelly and is covered by amnion. It supports and protects three blood vessels, namely one large umbilical vein carrying blood from the placenta to the fetus, and two umbilical arteries winding around the vein carrying deoxygenated blood from the fetus to the placenta (Fig. 3.19; see also 'The route of the blood').

The absence of a vessel may be associated with renal agenesis (absence of kidney).

Functions of the placenta

The placenta has *respiratory, nutritional, excretory, protective* and *endocrine* activities. It provides oxygen and removes carbon dioxide; it provides nutrients necessary for growth and removes waste products. It forms a barrier to certain

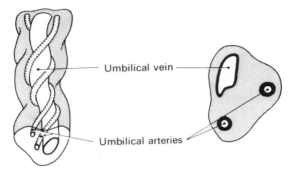

Fig. 3.19 The umbilical cord. Sideview and cross-section showing one umbilical vein with two umbilical arteries twisting spirally around it.

noxious materials such as bacteria. The placenta secretes oestrogens, progesterone and chorionic gonadotrophin.

Functions of the membranes and liquor

The membranes and liquor provide a medium in which the fetus can move and a cushion against knocks. An equable temperature is maintained, pressure is equalized and the cord itself is protected from excessive pressure.

4 Physiology and Management of Pregnancy

Before commencing the physiology and care of pregnancy there are several terms the nurse will need to understand.

Nullipara	A woman who has not had a pregnancy.
Primigravida	A woman pregnant for the first time.
Primipara	A woman at the end of her first labour and afterwards.
Multigravida	A woman pregnant for the second or subsequent time.
Multipara	A woman who has had more than one child.

PHYSIOLOGY OF PREGNANCY

Pregnancy is a time of emotional and physical change, during which the various systems of the body are fashioned for the role they will have to fulfil in supporting and eventually expelling the fetus. These changes can be considered under various headings.

Hormonal changes

Human chorionic gonadotrophin (HCG) When fertilization occurs, the HCG produced by the blastocyst causes the corpus luteum to persist and, because of this, the first sign of pregnancy is most usually amenorrhoea. The HCG reaches maximum production at about the 12th week of pregnancy, after which the corpus luteum gradually declines as the placenta develops and becomes active.

The HCG is excreted by the kidneys and can be detected in the urine from the early weeks of pregnancy; this is the basis of the biological and immunological pregnancy tests.

Oestrogens Oestrogens are produced first from the corpus luteum and subsequently from the placenta. Their effects are described in Chapter 2.

Oestrogens can be measured in the maternal serum as a test of placental function from about 30 weeks, or one particular oestrogen (oestriol) which is excreted in the mother's urine can be measured in a 24-hour collection of urine.

Progesterone The corpus luteum and, later, the placenta produce large quantities of progesterone and the general effects are described in Chapter 2.

During pregnancy, progesterone causes further proliferation of the uterine decidua which enables the embryo to embed, and it maintains the lining healthy during the pregnancy. Progesterone also relaxes all smooth muscle. In the uterus this prevents irritability and contractions which might expel the developing fetus. When the vascular tone is reduced the diastolic blood pressure is lowered and there is also an increased tendency to varicose veins and haemorrhoids. In the gastrointestinal tract, the reduction of muscle tone accounts for heartburn and constipation, and, in the ureters, relaxation and kinking may lead to stasis of urine and possibly urine infection.

Other endocrine glands, such as the anterior pituitary, thyroid and adrenal cortex, are enlarged. The increase in thyroid tissue accounts for the increased metabolic rate and contributes to the lability of mood in early pregnancy. The adrenocortical steroids do not increase markedly until after the first three months, this is nature's safeguard as cortico-steroids are one of the substances which can damage the fetus in the early weeks and cause abnormality. Steroids affect the fluid balance in pregnancy and may account for some of the weight gain.

The uterus

The uterus in its non-pregnant state measures 7.5 cm in length, 5 cm in width and 2.5 cm in depth, at term it is 30 cm long, 22.5 cm wide and 20 cm deep. It increases in weight from 60 to 700 g. This enlargement is accounted for by growth of existing muscle (hypertrophy) and the laying down of new muscle cells (hyperplasia). The most important factor is the thickness of the uterine wall: originally it is 1.25 cm and at the end of pregnancy 0.75 cm—this indicates tremendous growth. If the uterus merely stretched it would be paper thin and unable to do the work necessary to expel the fetus.

The uterus rises out of the pelvis at about the 12th week; the fundus reaches the level of the umbilicus at about 24 weeks and the xiphisternum at about 38 weeks (Fig. 4.1). The uterine tubes and ovaries are displaced out of the pelvis as the uterus enlarges. The cervix softens and becomes lilac in colour from the increased vascularity, and the cervical glands produce a tenacious mucus which forms a plug in the cervical canal and is known as operculum.

During late pregnancy and labour the uterus is described as having an upper and lower segment. The upper segment consists of the fundus and upper three-quarters of the body of the uterus. The lower segment develops from the isthmus and makes up the remaining one-quarter.

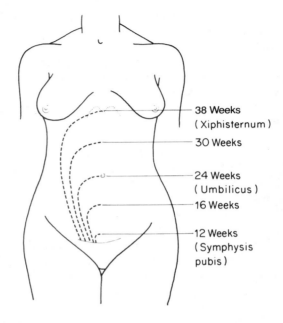

38 Weeks
(Xiphisternum)

30 Weeks

24 Weeks
(Umbilicus)

16 Weeks

12 Weeks
(Symphysis
pubis)

Fig. 4.1 The height of the uterus at different stages of gestation.

Skin changes

There are two main skin changes, caused by stretching or by pigmentation.

Changes caused by stretching can be seen on the anterior abdominal wall, in the breasts and the buttocks. Yellow elastic fibres in the skin rupture producing pinkish streaks known as striae gravidarum. After delivery these persist as silvery white scars. Similar markings may be seen in Cushing's syndrome (lineae distensae).

Changes caused by pigmentation are probably brought about by the increase of the anterior pituitary melanin-stimulating hormone. The nipples, the linea alba (the white line from umbilicus to pubis), the vulva and existing scars darken in colour. In some women a golden brown pigmentation, chloasma, may appear on the face. Many women are extremely conscious of this and it causes them distress, but they can be assured that it will disappear after delivery.

The breasts

The breasts enlarge as described in Chapter 10 and take on certain characteristic external signs. The woman experiences tingling sensations and sometimes discomfort in the early weeks of pregnancy.

Cardiovascular system

The enlarging uterus, placental site and breasts all require an increased blood supply, and the blood volume increases by about 25% from the 12th week. The consequent increased amount of work for the heart is of special significance when there is underlying cardiac disease.

There is a smaller increase in red blood cells and haemoglobin compared with the increase in blood volume, so haemodilution occurs. The plasma proteins are also decreased, which may contribute towards oedema which is often seen in late pregnancy.

The blood pressure normally falls slightly, especially during the second trimester of pregnancy.

Urinary tract

The work of the kidneys increases with the increased blood flow. The renal threshold for sugar is lowered so that glycosuria may occur without the blood glucose level being raised. The bladder is displaced in very early and late pregnancy, and the ureters are relaxed and dilated, causing frequency of micturition, and can kink (Fig. 4.2).

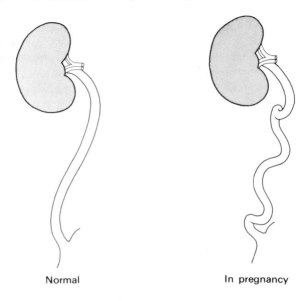

Normal   In pregnancy

Fig. 4.2 Diagram showing relaxation of the ureter in pregnancy.

Weight

The weight increase during pregnancy is not only from the growing fetus, but also from maternal tissues. The total weight gain in pregnancy should not exceed 13 kg, and at term this is distributed approximately as follows.

Storage of fat and protein	4.0 kg
Fetus	3.3 kg
Water and electrolytes	1.5 kg
Liquor	1.4 kg
Breasts	1.0 kg
Uterus	0.7 kg
Placenta	0.6 kg

Total 12.5 kg

Emotional changes

At all times of major changes in the hormones there is emotional instability; but quite apart from hormonal influences, a woman experiences the emotional effects of the substantial changes in her whole lifestyle which having a baby involves.

The atmosphere in some antenatal clinics can be so clinical that patients feel ashamed to confess the emotional part of pregnancy: but nurses in the clinic should allow the expression of these very real and normal feelings.

Because the outcome of a pregnancy is unknown, the woman may experience wide fluctuations in mood, from a tremendous confidence about the healthy baby she longs for, to tearful dread that old wives' tales may be true. She may be laughing one moment and in tears the next: even the most placid women may be irritable or uneasy. This bewilders the husband if he does not understand what is happening and any marriage stresses may become highlighted.

During the first trimester, the patient has the initial impact of the news of her pregnancy. This is often one of sheer delight, but the nurse cannot presume that this is the case. A woman's reaction depends on factors such as whether the pregnancy was unplanned or long awaited, or on whether she is married and how her husband reacts. She may have a mixture of emotions: for example, if she has had a miscarriage previously, she may be delighted yet simultaneously apprehensive about the present pregnancy. If she is unmarried, she may want to escape from her unwelcome plight by having the pregnancy terminated, yet also feel guilty about destroying the life of her baby.

Although the nurse may feel helpless amidst such strong emotions, she can often help by enabling the patient to talk and thereby formulate her emotions, perhaps for the first time.

During the second trimester a mother becomes increasingly

conscious that she is pregnant. She not only looks pregnant, but also she can feel the baby moving; and so emotionally she begins to expect a baby. This is exciting to a woman who is pleased about the pregnancy, but only reinforces any resentment or fear for one who finds it difficult to accept what is happening within her.

During the last three months a woman is physically tired, she becomes increasingly aware of her inescapable responsibilities as a parent, and her thoughts are often dominated by the labour which looms ahead. The nurse can help by giving practical advice about rest and sleep, parentcraft education, and preparation for labour (pages 52–56); but of prime importance is her willingness to give the emotional support that each patient needs, especially if the husband does not give this. Confidence in the nurses is built up when the patient is given time in which to express her fears and ask questions.

ANTENATAL CLINICS

Every woman in the United Kingdom is entitled to antenatal care without payment. Its aims are to maintain or even improve the mother's health, so that she may deliver a healthy baby; to detect abnormalities so as to give help as early as possible and prevent further complications; to educate the mother, and to establish good rapport between mother and midwife or doctor.

Women are encouraged to seek antenatal care early in the pregnancy, but this encouragement must be backed up by the right atmosphere in the clinic. All too often clinics are so crowded, rushed, or humiliating, that patients prefer not to come. It is essential that each patient is given respect and privacy at all times, and that she knows that she can neither be overheard nor overlooked. In short, she should be made to feel a person, not just a name amongst many others (see Fig. 4.3).

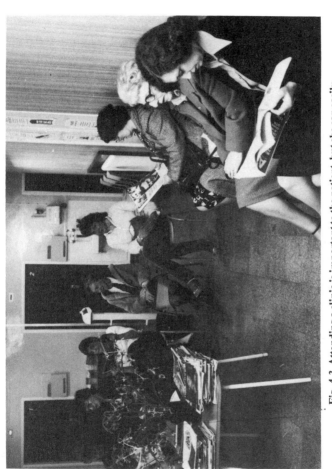

Fig. 4.3 Attending a clinic is important to the patient, but she can easily feel depersonalized as 'just another in the queue'. The nurse must give special attention to each one.

The nurse has to adapt her manner in antenatal clinic to patients' different expectations of her. Patients at an antenatal clinic are not ill, therefore on the whole they are not grateful for being made better, in the same way as sick patients are in other clinics. Antenatal patients are notably interested in events, since they find themselves taking part in the fascinating miracle of new life: this opens the patient's mind so she welcomes appropriate advice and discussion.

The first visit

The first visit involves a thorough examination early in pregnancy in order to assess a baseline from which progress can be measured during the course of the pregnancy. This is usually before 12 weeks gestation.

Examination of the patient at this clinic is similar to gynaecological examination (see Chapter 20). The three parts of the examination are adapted to obstetrics as outlined below.

Taking the history The patient's history is extremely important because it may suggest specific areas of need by revealing any previous abnormalities which may recur or affect the pregnancy. Each aspect is summarized here, but the nurse should expand the history in any aspect relevant to the wellbeing of mother and baby.

Social history The correct name, address, age and religion are taken down, the first to facilitate correct recording, and the age because it may have some bearing on the care to be given, for instance an older woman having her first baby may need to be seen more often. The name of the patient's own doctor is also noted so that he may be informed of her progress. The duration of marriage may give two helpful pointers: first, the unmarried mother who will need special help and advice, and second the woman who has had great difficulty in becoming pregnant.

Medical history The medical history may reveal the need for special care during the pregnancy, for example conditions such as cardiac disease, diabetes, or tuberculosis (Chapter 6). Some diseases leave permanent damage, such as acute rheumatism, chorea, or diphtheria. Any operations, especially those which involved the genital tract or which left a scar on the uterus, should be noted, with any accidents involving the pelvis or previous blood transfusions.

Family history Inquiries are made about hereditary diseases such as diabetes, hypertension, tuberculosis or mental illness, and whether there is a history of multiple pregnancy in either family.

Menstrual history The frequency and duration of menstruation are important because conception is calculated as occurring 14 days prior to the next expected menstrual period. In a woman with infrequent periods the expected date of delivery must be calculated accordingly.

Expected date of delivery (EDD) The EDD is important because at every antenatal examination the size of the uterus can be compared with the size expected by the gestational dates. Later in the pregnancy it may become necessary to stop premature labour or to induce labour if the baby is very overdue, and these decisions can only be based on an EDD.

The EDD is estimated by adding seven days to the first day of the last menstrual period (LMP), and adding nine months, making a total of 40 weeks or 280 days.

Example

LMP	5.4.82	EDD	12.1.83
LMP	29.7.82	EDD	5.5.83

The EDD is only approximate and may vary by ten days either way, which is important to try to impress on the patient because she will worry a great deal when the stated day comes and goes and labour does not commence.

Obstetric history A clear summary of any previous pregnancies and miscarriages is important, noting particularly the duration of pregnancy, complications, the length of labour and type of delivery, and any complication following. Information about the baby should be added, to include sex and weight of the baby, whether it was breast- or bottle-fed, and if it is still alive.

The patient is usually grateful for explanations as to why she is being asked so many questions, and for reassurance that they are indeed relevant to the management of her pregnancy. History taking should thus not be an inquisition in which a patient fumbles for the right answer, but rather it becomes a two-way communication between nurse and patient, full of helpful explanations to one another.

Physical examination When the history is complete, a routine physical examination of the patient is made. The duties of the nurse are described on page 242.

In the first examination, the height and weight of the patient are recorded.

Haematological examination Specimens of blood are taken for blood grouping, the Rhesus factor and haemoglobin estimation. Wassermann–Kahn tests are carried out to exclude syphilis. In immigrant women from West Africa and the West Indies, tests to identify sickle cells are included.

Examination of urine Urine is tested at every visit for the presence of protein, glucose and ketoacids, none of which should be present, although glycosuria can occur with the lowered renal threshold (see page 35). Proteinuria may indicate pre-eclampsia and glycosuria diabetes mellitus. In some clinics it is routine to carry out a bacteriological examination on the first specimen to exclude subclinical urinary infection.

The urine sample taken at each visit empties the patient's bladder to facilitate general medical examination.

General medical examination To exclude any underlying disease, general medical examination includes examination of the cardiovascular system and recording of the blood pressure. Due to the physiological changes, the latter is a little lower than one might expect and anything above 130/90 may be due to pathological causes.

Examination of the breasts The breasts are examined for changes which might confirm pregnancy and to determine if breast-feeding is likely to be easy or difficult.

Examination of the abdomen An abdominal examination will reveal the height of the fundus and will help to confirm the expected date of delivery (see page 45–46).

Examination of the pelvis A vaginal examination may be carried out at the first visit or later in pregnancy. Early on, it confirms the diagnosis of pregnancy and gives the obstetrician an idea of the pelvic shape and size. A more valuable examination is carried out at about the 36th week of pregnancy when it is possible to feel the fetal head in relation to the maternal pelvis and assess if it is likely to pass through.

Examination of the legs The legs are examined for equality of length and muscle wasting which might indicate alteration of pelvic shape. Signs of oedema should be elicited by pressing over the tibia just above the external malleolus and observing if pitting occurs. Finally, varicose veins should be noted and supported if present.

Discussion The observations from all of the above examinations are recorded, both on the patient's medical notes and also on her 'cooperation card'. The latter is given to the patient for her to carry around with her all the time so that whichever doctor or midwife attends her, she can show this summary of her history and present pregnancy.

The management of the pregnancy can be planned with the patient, for example special tests (see pages 48–51) or appropriate advice given (see pages 52–56). Decisions will be made about the place of her confinement and whether her care will be undertaken by the GP alone or shared between hospital and GP. Any plans for future management may need to be changed, depending on the progress of the pregnancy. Once again, it is important to bear in mind that the patient has the right to be involved in any decisions, and indeed she should be encouraged to take an active interest in the well-being of herself and her baby.

Subsequent visits

Visits to the clinic usually begin at monthly intervals until about 28 weeks, then every two weeks to the 36th week, and weekly thereafter. These visits may be made more frequent if there are any abnormalities. The haemoglobin level is re-estimated at intervals and in the case of the Rhesus-negative woman the blood is examined for antibody production (see page 168). At 16 weeks, serum alpha fetoprotein (SAFP) can be measured: high levels are associated with open neural tube defects.

At each subsequent visit, the urine is tested, blood pressure and weight are recorded, the ankles examined for oedema, and an abdominal examination is carried out.

The abdominal examination

The woman is arranged on the examination couch with not more than two pillows and the abdomen exposed from beneath the breasts to the symphysis pubis. The examiner stands on the patient's right.

There are three parts to this examination: inspection, palpation and auscultation.

Inspection The shape and size of the abdomen are looked at. If muscles are young and firm as in the primigravida, they fit firmly over the uterus which appears rather egg shaped with the broad end uppermost. In the multigravida it is rounder and more lax. Scars, striae and fetal movements are also noted.

Palpation Palpation determines several things, and for the student nurse this is one of the most difficult tasks. Until now she will not have used her hands to effect a clinical diagnosis. Hands must be warm and finger-nails short to avoid hurting the patient.

The *height of the fundus* (Fig. 4.1) is determined with the ulnar border of the left hand, and should agree with the period of amenorrhoea.

Now, using both hands flat on the abdominal wall in a manoeuvre which will be demonstrated by the midwife, various details are determined.

The *lie* relates the spine of the fetus to the maternal spine and may be longitudinal, oblique or transverse (Fig. 4.4).

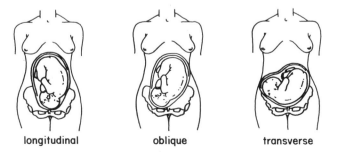

longitudinal   oblique   transverse

Fig. 4.4 Diagrams showing the lie of the fetus.

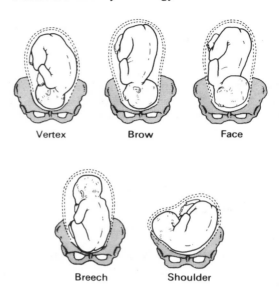

Vertex   Brow   Face

Breech   Shoulder

Fig. 4.5 Five types of presentation.

The *presentation* is the part of the fetus that is lowest in the birth canal and may be a vertex, face, brow, breech or shoulder (Fig. 4.5).

The *position* relates the denominator (a given point on the fetus) to a particular part of the pelvis in order to describe which way the fetus is facing. The denominator is the occiput in a vertex presentation, or the sacrum in a breech presentation, or the mentum (chin) in a face presentation. For example, if the occiput is resting towards the mother's left, anteriorly, the position is described as left occipito-anterior (Fig. 4.6).

The *attitude* relates the fetal head and limbs to its body and may be fully flexed, poorly flexed, or extended (Fig. 4.7).

Engagement means that the biparietal diameter has passed through the pelvic brim (Fig. 4.8). In the primigravida it occurs at about 36 weeks but in multiparae later, sometimes

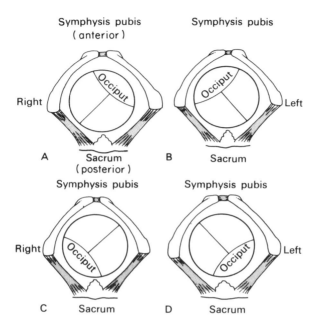

**Fig. 4.6 Diagrammatic representation of the positions of the fetal skull.
A. Left occipito-anterior. B. Right occipito-anterior. C. Right
occipito-posterior. D. Left occipito-posterior.**

during labour. Engagement is important because it proves
that the fetal head is not too big to enter the pelvic brim and
that vaginal delivery should be feasible.

The patients refer to engagement as lightening because of
the sense of lightness they feel when the pressure lessens on
the diaphragm.

Auscultation The fetal heart can be heard by means of a
Pinard's (fetal) stethoscope (Fig. 4.9) through the abdominal
wall. It is heard below the level of the umbilicus in cephalic

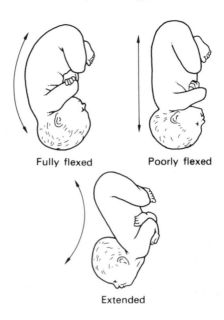

Fully flexed   Poorly flexed

Extended

Fig. 4.7 The attitude of the fetus.

(head) presentations and above the umbilicus in podalic (breech) presentations.

The mother should always be reassured when her baby's heart beat has been heard. If the student nurse is not well practised at listening, it is fairer to explain this to the mother beforehand, who may otherwise fear that her baby has died.

Special tests

At any time, special tests may be carried out to monitor the fetus, the aim of these being to detect earliest signs of any deviation from normal and to prevent development of complications to the mother or the fetus. These tests are a

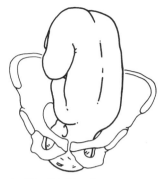

Fig. 4.8 Engagement of the fetal head.

helpful complement to, but never a substitute for, clinical judgement by inspection, palpation, and auscultation.

Ultrasound scan See page 115.

Placental function tests The wellbeing of the fetus can be assessed by measuring levels of placental hormones in the mother: poor placental function is detrimental to the fetus. There are two main tests:

   urinary oestriol—measured in a 24-hour collection of urine

   human placental lactogen—measured in the mother's serum.

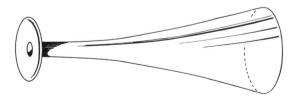

Fig. 4.9 Pinard's fetal stethoscope.

Fetal movements chart Research has shown that infrequent fetal movements are associated with an unhealthy fetus. The mother is asked to count the number of times she feels her baby move per morning, and to consult her doctor if she feels very few or no movements at all on any day.

X-rays X-rays are only harmful to the fetus in the early weeks of pregnancy. Abdominal x-rays may be taken in late pregnancy to show the position of the fetus or fetuses, and to measure the relationship of the fetal head to the maternal pelvis (pelvimetry).

Amniocentesis Amniocentesis is the withdrawal of liquor from around the fetus. This liquor contains cells shed by the fetus which can be cultured and examined, for example:

1. to detect chromosomal abnormality
2. to check liquor alpha fetoprotein (this is more accurate than SAFP)
3. to test for lung maturity prior to early induction of labour.

Cardiotocograph Continuous monitoring of fetal heart rate can be printed on a graph by a special monitor. One hour's continuous monitoring shows patterns of the fetal heart rate which can be interpreted by the obstetrician. This can be even more accurate after rupture of membranes because a scalp electrode can provide a fetal ECG when intensive monitoring is required.

The mother may feel quite overwhelmed by the machinery, so the nurse must remember that her duty is to care for the patient and not merely to observe a machine (Fig. 4.10).

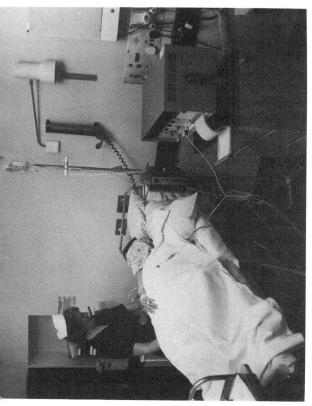

Fig. 4.10 Patients in labour can misconstrue help as interference. The nurse should show that she is caring for the patient and not merely observing a machine.

ADVICE TO THE PREGNANT WOMAN

In the antenatal period women are very receptive to advice and there is a wonderful opportunity for health education. Most of the advice is given by the midwife in private discussion or to small groups at parentcraft classes.

Hygienic care

It is as essential in pregnancy as at any other time to keep the body clean, especially the area of the external genitalia as vaginal secretion is likely to be heavier. In late pregnancy the woman may find it easier to kneel in the bath and also to have someone attend to her toe-nails: she cannot see her feet easily, far less reach them.

Clothing

Most expectant mothers naturally choose the right sort of clothes for pregnancy, to look attractive yet feel comfortable and free from restrictions around the waist.

Many women find support tights helpful, especially if they have varicose veins. Any constrictive garments, such as elasticated stockings, should be avoided because they restrict venous return.

Advice should be given about brassieres, even if the woman does not intend to breast-feed. The breasts should be supported well, such that they do not sag with the extra weight (1 kg). The straps should be wide so that they do not cut into the shoulders.

Shoes should have a stable, broad-based heel but need not be flat.

Exercise

Fresh air and exercise should be taken each day as this improves circulation and muscle tone, but violent unaccustomed exercise should be avoided. Special exercises and relaxation may be taught at parentcraft classes.

Rest

Exercise must be balanced with rest because the whole basal metabolic rate is increased during pregnancy and a woman can easily become tired. An afternoon rest is desirable but not always possible if the woman is still working, but should be encouraged in late pregnancy, when the night's rest is disturbed by frequency of micturition and the fetus kicking. Long journeys by car or train should be avoided in late pregnancy as the jolting could cause labour to commence in some people. The doctor is best consulted before an aeroplane flight is embarked upon.

Diet

The idea of eating for two is quite false, as far as quantity is concerned. The needs of the fetus must be supplied, however, so mothers should pay special attention to the quality of food.

Good first-class protein, meat, fish, eggs and dairy produce should be taken and at least one pint of milk per day. Carbohydrates and fats should be limited as they are inclined to increase weight. Green vegetables, fresh fruit and roughage-containing foods such as wholemeal bread and certain cereals will often assist in the prevention of constipation, and so avoid the injudicious use of aperients.

Drugs

It is not possible to prove that any drug is completely harmless in pregnancy, but some are definitely harmful. All patients should be advised to consult the doctor or midwife about any drugs.

Smoking is a form of drug taking and causes placental insufficiency and smaller babies. Heavy smokers should be warned that they are 'smoking for two'. Even small amounts of alcohol are thought to affect the fetus.

Teeth

Teeth should be examined regularly during pregnancy because gingival tissues are affected by the hormones of pregnancy presdisposing to dental caries. Patients should be reminded that dental treatment is free during pregnancy.

Breasts and breast-feeding

The mother's intentions for feeding her baby should be discussed before delivery and, if she wants to breast-feed, she can make certain preparations.

The breasts should be kept clean, and after washing they can be dried using a turkish towel whose friction improves the circulation. The breasts exude a secretion called colostrum, which dries and forms crusts on the nipples and will cause soreness if not removed when washing. During the last few weeks of pregnancy a small amount of this colostrum can be expressed from the breasts. This accustoms the patient to handling her breasts, although it is thought that valuable antibodies may be lost if this is overdone.

Individual advice will be required if the nipples are flat or retracted; they may be improved by gently pulling them out with the thumb and first finger, or Woolwich shells may be worn for a few hours daily (Fig. 4.11).

Sexual intercourse

There is no medical contraindication to sexual intercourse during pregnancy, except occasionally for patients with a history of miscarriage or premature labour.

Parentcraft teaching

Many prospective parents benefit from classes which teach basic skills of parentcraft, such as bathing and dressing,

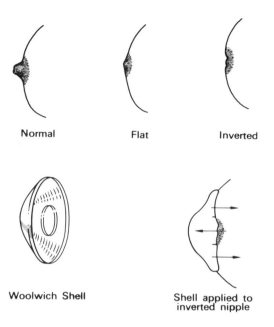

Normal   Flat   Inverted

Woolwich Shell

Shell applied to
inverted nipple

**Fig. 4.11 Diagram of the types of nipple. Woolwich breast shell applied
to the inverted nipple.**

sterilization of bottles and discussion about the layette,
breast- and bottle-feeding (see Chapter 11). Details of these
classes should be displayed prominently in antenatal clinics
and health centres so as to capture the interest. The
atmosphere should be friendly and informal; groups should
be small and a cup of tea together may break down many
barriers.

Relaxation classes and psychoprophylaxis
Teaching about relaxation, psychoprophylaxis and psycho-
physical preparation for labour is often incorporated into

parentcraft classes, but some special classes are also run, such as by the National Childbirth Trust. Their purpose is to prepare the mother for labour, by teaching specific exercises by which she can participate actively in labour. Voluntary muscles thereby assist, rather than antagonize, the work of involuntary muscles. Women are taught something of the physiology of labour, how to breathe at the various stages, and the best way to relax in between contractions.

All the methods differ slightly but they give the patient information and confidence which help to dispel her fear and anxiety. It is essential that the same method is continued during labour, otherwise both patient and nurse become confused. Fathers are encouraged to attend as often as possible.

Financial benefits

Each mother should be advised as to which financial benefits she is entitled (see Chapter 14).

FURTHER READING

HEARDMAN, H. & EBNER, M. (1975) *Relaxation and Exercise for Natural Childbirth*. Edinburgh, London and New York: Churchill Livingstone.

5 Bleeding during Pregnancy

Bleeding from the genital tract is considered in two groups: bleeding before the 28th week (threatened abortion) and bleeding after the 28th week (antepartum haemorrhage). The dividing line of 28 weeks is the age at which the fetus is said to be legally viable: that is, capable of an existence apart from its mother. In reality, with improving neonatal facilities, many babies survive before the age of 28 weeks and there is current pressure to change the legal definition such that viability is from 24 weeks gestation.

BLEEDING BEFORE THE 28TH WEEK

Ectopic gestation

Ectopic gestation is a pregnancy occurring outside the uterine cavity—usually the uterine tube (Fig. 5.1). It occurs in about 1 in 150 pregnancies and carries the risk of maternal death from severe haemorrhage.

Tubal pregnancy arises when some factor has slowed the progress of the ovum through the tube (refer to Chapter 27), as a result of fibrosis, congenital abnormality of the tube, or if the ovum migrates to the opposite tube across the pelvic cavity.

The muscle of the tube, having no submucosa, is easily invaded by the trophoblast, which soon penetrates an arteriole or artery. Once bleeding begins, the villus is unable to plug the rent, and high arteriolar pressure forces blood out which strips the rest of the villi from their anchorage. In 65% of cases the ovum separates completely and aborts spontaneously,

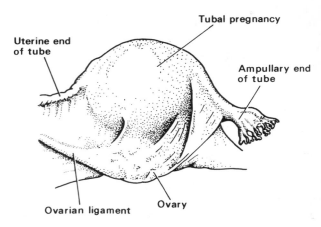

Fig. 5.1 Tubal pregnancy.

but there may be complications such as haematosalpinx or tubal mole; or the tube may rupture (Fig. 5.2) and cause an acute abdominal emergency.

Signs and symptoms There is usually a history of amenorrhoea with signs of early pregnancy, although if implantation occurred at the isthmus it may rupture before menstruation is late.

The main symptom is a sudden attack of one-sided lower abdominal pain associated with vaginal bleeding. If the tube ruptures there are signs of collapse and shock, with pallor, cold clammy skin, rapid pulse, faintness and vomiting. Pain may be referred to the shoulder if blood tracks to the diaphragm and stimulates the phrenic nerve.

On examination there is a brownish discharge, known as 'prune juice discharge'. Vaginal examination reveals extreme tenderness over the gravid tube and in the pouch of Douglas. If there is peritoneal irritation, there is muscle guarding and, later, a slight pyrexia.

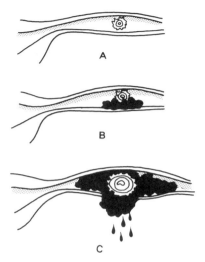

Fig. 5.2 A: Fertilized ovum in a uterine tube;
B: Separation of the chorionic villi;
C: Rupture of the tube.

Diagnosis is confirmed by laparoscopy, which may be necessary to differentiate from acute appendicitis or salpingitis; but ectopic pregnancy is an acute surgical emergency requiring immediate treatment.

Treatment An intravenous infusion is set up followed by blood transfusion, and the patient is taken to theatre with the minimum of preparation. If laparoscopy reveals tubal pregnancy, a laparotomy is performed to ligate bleeding points and remove the tube.

The patient's condition improves as soon as bleeding is controlled. Intravenous fluids are discontinued once the blood pressure has returned to normal. The patient rapidly feels better physically, but this is the time when she feels the impact of the significance of losing the pregnancy, especially if the baby was longed for. Unfortunately there is a 10% chance of a further ectopic pregnancy in the other tube.

ABORTION

Abortion means the cessation of pregnancy before the 28th week. The terms miscarriage and abortion are synonymous although the word abortion is seldom used to and by the patient because there is a prevalent but mistaken idea that abortion implies criminal interference. Abortion is the commonest cause of early bleeding and is known to occur in at least one in seven pregnancies. Abortion constitutes the greatest cause of maternal death in the United Kingdom.

Women react in different ways to abortion. Some consider pregnancy only in relation to their own bodies and disregard the existence of the growing fetus within. Others are more aware of the life which has been lost, seeing it as being precious, and they tend to mourn more than those who

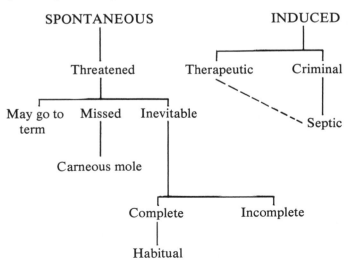

suppress thoughts of that life, however primitive. The nuse
suppress thoughts of that life, however primitive. The nurse
must be aware of the very individual reaction and consequent
needs of each patient. Some patients want to keep their
feelings private, or share them only with the husband, whilst
others seek positive support or guidance from the nurses.
Having assessed these needs once, the nurse should constantly
be alert to see change as the patient comes to terms
psychologically with what has happened physically.

Abortion can be divided into spontaneous and induced.

SPONTANEOUS ABORTION

Threatened abortion

A threatened abortion is the term given for any vaginal
bleeding which occurs before the 28th week, before the
outcome of the bleeding is known. There may be slight
abdominal cramp or backache but the cervical os is closed
and the membranes remain intact (Fig. 5.3).

Treatment The patient is confined to bed until bleeding
ceases, when she will gradually be allowed up. All pads are

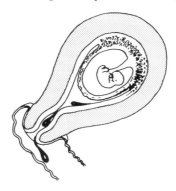

Fig. 5.3 Threatened abortion.

saved to assess the amount of blood loss. Early morning specimens of urine are sent for pregnancy testing (HCG measurements) each day.

This is a time of great uncertainty for the patient, whose hopes fluctuate every time bleeding diminishes or increases. She will be anxious to be informed of the results of tests and examinations because the outcome of a threatened abortion is unknown. Many pregnancies continue to term, but in some bleeding continues and abortion becomes inevitable, and in others the fetus dies and a mole forms.

Inevitable abortion

Abortion is inevitable once the cervix has begun to dilate. Bleeding becomes more profuse and can be severe. In early pregnancy, HCG measurements fall markedly and products of conception may be seen at the cervical os. In later pregnancy, intermittent pain is felt, and these contractions continue strongly enough to expel the fetus.

If the whole ovum, fetus and chorionic tissue are expelled this is a *complete abortion*, but if some of the products of conception are retained it is an *incomplete abortion*. In early pregnancy abortion is often incomplete because separation of the chorion is not easy from the poorly developed perforation layer of the decidua.

Treatment The doctor should be summoned because blood loss can be severe, requiring emergency help. All pads should be saved for inspection as the small fetus might be confused with blood clot, and it is important to ascertain if the products of conception have been completely expelled.

If the abortion is complete and bleeding has ceased, the patient can remain at home, but if it is incomplete she should be taken to theatre as soon as possible for evacuation of retained products of conception (see Dilatation and Curretage, pages 320–321). If blood loss is heavy, an oxytocic drug will be given, and cross-matched blood will be transfused. Pethidine hydrochloride 100 mg may be given to ease the pain and calm the patient.

The nurse's responsibility is to give support and reassurance to the patient whilst she carries out observations of the pulse, blood pressure and vaginal loss. Once the abortion is complete she should ensure that adequate care is given to vulval toilet: the vulval area should be washed or swabbed at least twice daily. The patient will be discharged home the day after abortion is complete.

Missed abortion

A missed abortion, or carneous mole, occurs when the embryo dies but remains in utero, the gestational sac separates and becomes surrounded by organized blood clot (Fig. 5.4). The signs and symptoms of pregnancy disappear, but amenorrhoea persists and there is usually a brown vaginal discharge.

The amenorrhoea often prevents the patient from suspecting that anything is wrong, especially if there is no discharge.

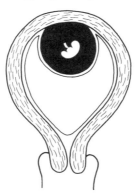

Fig. 5.4 Missed abortion (carneous mole) showing the ovum surrounded by a blood clot.

However, on examination the uterus is smaller than the size expected by dates; urinary HCG levels are low, and the diagnosis may be confirmed by ultrasound scan.

Treatment Treatment is usually given because most women find the idea of a dead fetus in utero very distressing. If surgical intervention is not desirable, an oxytocic drug may be given in an effort to make the uterus contract and expel its contents; otherwise the patient is taken to theatre for dilatation and curettage (see pages 320–321).

A patient may take longer to come to terms with a missed abortion since she has not experienced the fresh blood loss and she may find it hard to believe that the fetus has in fact died. The nurse should be gentle in her explanations, allowing the patient time to assimilate what is happening to her.

Habitual abortion

The term habitual abortion is used when there have been three or more consecutive abortions. This causes much distress to the woman and her husband; with the news of each further pregnancy comes a mixture of hope and dread that this too will end in grief.

Treatment Careful investigations are undertaken to try to detect abnormality such as congenital malformation, systemic disease or karyotypic abnormality. Often, however, no cause is found and treatment is empirical.

When the patient becomes pregnant again, she is admitted to hospital for strict bedrest around the time when abortion has previously occurred. Hormone therapy is sometimes given, such as progesterone (Primulot Depot 250 mg twice weekly) or HCG. A Shirodkar suture is usually inserted if there is any cervical incompetence (see Chapter 8).

INDUCED ABORTION

Induced abortions are divided into therapeutic and criminal.

Therapeutic abortion

Termination of pregnancy is legal in the United Kingdom under the Abortion Act of 1967, provided that two doctors, each having examined the patient, sign a notification to the Medical Officer of Health stating that the continuation of pregnancy involves a *greater* risk than termination:

1. to the life of the mother
2. to the physical or mental health of the mother
3. to the physical or mental health of existing child(ren), or
4. if there is a substantial risk of serious physical or mental abnormality in the baby.

Pregnancy can be terminated either surgically or medically.

Surgical methods Before ten weeks the uterus is evacuated using suction via a plastic (Karman) curette. This is done under general or local anaesthetic and the patient is discharged on the same or the following day.

When the pregnancy is more advanced, abdominal hysterotomy may be performed. These surgical methods carry the risks of local trauma and those of any general anaesthetic.

Medical methods Medical induction is performed after about 14 weeks, using prostaglandins or intra-amniotic instillations (such as hypertonic saline). Prostaglandins are injected continuously into the extra-amniotic sac, or into the amniotic cavity or, occasionally, intravenously. Medical induction of abortion is more unpleasant to the patient, who is unlikely to forget the experience.

Criminal abortion

This is the evacuation of contents of the uterus by unauthorized persons and is an offence punishable by law. It occurs much less frequently since the Abortion Act of 1967. Criminal abortion frequently leads to a tragic sequence of events. The methods employed may cause sudden death from haemorrhage or air embolus. Because of the lack of asepsis, infection readily occurs (see Septic Abortion), and may lead to chronic invalidism, or salpingitis which results in blocked tubes and the inability to conceive at a later date.

The nurse is a vulnerable member of the community because she may be asked for advice, or for help when bleeding occurs. She should never do anything except on the instruction of a doctor or she herself may be liable to prosecution. Once a patient is admitted to hospital, however, the nurse's duty is to care for her as thoroughly as for all her patients.

Septic abortion

Septic abortion results from incomplete abortion, when retained products of conception become infected, or from sepsis introduced during therapeutic or criminal abortion. The patient has pyrexia, tachycardia, malaise and there may be signs of pelvic peritonitis.

On examination, the uterus is tender and vaginal loss is offensive and profuse. In severe cases there is a danger of septicaemia, renal failure and death.

The patient should be isolated, a high vaginal swab taken and sent for bacteriological examination. Antibiotics are given and blood transfusion may be necessary. Some obstetricians perform curettage under general anaesthetic, although there is a risk of rupturing the uterus.

Nursing care is as for severe salpingitis (see Chapter 27).

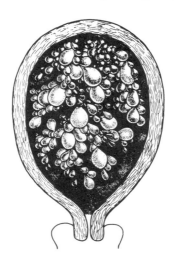

Fig. 5.5 A hydatidiform mole.

HYDATIDIFORM MOLE

A hydatidiform mole is a mass of vesicles resembling a bunch of grapes which are the result of abnormal development of the chorionic villi. The fetus is not in evidence (Fig. 5.5).

Signs and symptoms The normal signs of pregnancy tend to be exaggerated—there is excessive nausea and vomiting, the uterus is larger than dates, and there may be early signs of pre-eclampsia. Because of the tremendous chorionic activity, the output of HCG is excessive, which is a diagnostic feature, when at great dilution the urine still gives a positive pregnancy test. The patient has not felt fetal movements and she may complain of intermittent small amounts of vaginal bleeding.

On examination the uterus feels soft and doughy, there are

no palpable fetal parts and the fetal heart is not heard. Diagnosis may be confirmed by ultrasound scan.

Treatment The uterus is emptied as soon as a diagnosis is made. Fortunately this often occurs spontaneously, leaving a relatively small amount to be evacuated by operation. The evacuation is performed vaginally if the uterus is not too large (up to the size of 16 weeks pregnancy), otherwise an abdominal hysterotomy has to be performed. Intravenous oxytocin may also be used.

The dangers of spontaneous expulsion or operation are haemorrhage and sepsis.

It is important to make sure that the uterus is empty, and to keep the patient under observation for some years by repeated urine tests for HCG measurement because of the danger that she may develop choriocarcinoma.

Choriocarcinoma One per cent of patients subsequently develop a *choriocarcinoma* which is a highly malignant tumour, death occurring within a few months. The immunological tests for pregnancy become strongly positive again and bleeding begins. As the growth infiltrates the uterus and vagina, pain increases, and spread occurs by the bloodstream to lungs, liver and brain.

Treatment of choriocarcinoma consists of high doses of methotrexate (an antifolic acid agent which disorganizes cell metabolism) given with 6-mercaptopurine or nitrogen mustard for three to five days. The course may be repeated after a week's rest. Side-effects are common and serious and patients are usually admitted to a specialist unit. A total hysterectomy with the removal of tubes and ovaries should be carried out if bleeding continues, or in patients whose families are complete.

BLEEDING AFTER THE 28TH WEEK

Antepartum haemorrhage

Antepartum haemorrhage is defined as bleeding from the genital tract after the 28th week, and before delivery of the fetus. Since the type of antepartum haemorrhage cannot be determined immediately, all patients must be admitted to hospital, however small the loss has been, because bleeding may recur at any time with serious complications endangering the lives of both mother and baby.

There are three main causes of antepartum haemorrhage: placenta praevia, placental abruption, and incidental causes.

Placenta praevia

If the placenta lies wholly or partially in the lower uterine segment, it is inevitable that as the lower segment stretches during the latter weeks of pregnancy there will be some separation of the placenta and therefore bleeding from the placental site. The greater the amount of placenta covering the internal os the greater will be the blood loss.

Placenta praevia is classified according to four types (Fig. 5.6).

Type I   The placenta is mainly in the upper segment but encroaching on the lower segment.

Type II   The placenta reaches to but does not cover the internal os.

Type III   The placenta covers the internal os when it is closed but not completely when it is dilated.

Type IV   The placenta completely covers the internal os.

Signs and symptoms The patient gives a history of painless vaginal bleeding, usually around 30–32 weeks gestation. On examination the lie of the fetus is often unstable, and the presenting part cannot be made to engage in

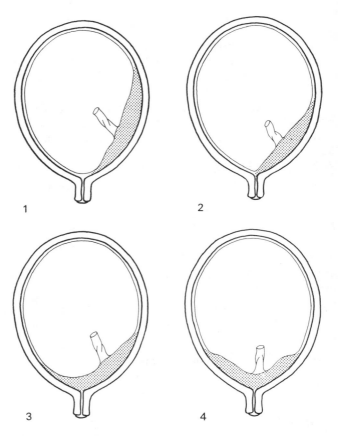

Fig. 5.6 Placenta praevia, types I to IV.

the pelvis. Diagnosis may be confirmed by ultrasound scan whereby the placenta can be localized.

Placental abruption ('accidental' haemorrhage)

Placental abruption is bleeding from complete or partial separation of a normally sited placenta. Bleeding is usually

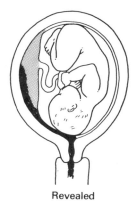

Revealed

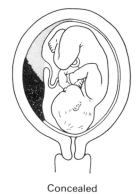

Concealed

Fig. 5.7 Placental abruption.

seen *per vaginam* ('revealed' haemorrhage), but sometimes the blood does not escape from the uterus ('concealed' haemorrhage—Fig. 5.7).

Signs and symptoms Placental abruption is a grave emergency because loss of placental function is fatal to the fetus, and maternal haemorrhage and associated shock or coagulation disorders can rapidly lead to maternal death.

There is a history of severe abdominal pain, usually accompanied by vaginal bleeding. On examination the uterus is hard, like wood, to the touch. Depending on the severity of the haemorrhage, the patient may show signs of shock and the fetal heartbeat may be absent. The urine may contain protein from renal damage.

Placental abruption is commonly associated with pre-eclampsia or hypertension.

Incidental causes

Bleeding can occur from local lesions of the cervix or vagina, such as a polyp, erosion, vaginitis or (rarely) carcinoma.

However, the cause of antepartum haemorrhage is often unknown.

Management of antepartum haemorrhage The aim of management is to protect the life of the mother and then the fetus. The actual treatment depends on the cause, the amount of bleeding and the period of gestation.

The temperature, pulse, blood pressure and blood loss should be observed and recorded. Urine is tested for protein and the abdominal girth is measured because this increases with concealed placental abruption. Blood should be cross-matched for transfusion if necessary, and a sedative may be given to help the patient to rest. She and her husband should be given adequate explanation of what is happening to her, without being alarmed, because they are naturally anxious to hear about their baby.

Ultrasound scan is performed to identify the position of the placenta, in order to establish the diagnosis. If the cause of bleeding is still uncertain, the patient remains in hospital until about 38 weeks gestation, during which time the well-being of the fetus should be monitored, and placental function tests are particularly important (see pages 48–51). This prolonged stay in hospital can lead to boredom and calls for skilled nursing care whereby the time can be used constructively, such as by giving parentcraft education and occupational therapy (see pages 151–155).

A Rhesus-negative mother should have blood tests for Rhesus antibodies and Kleihauer's test, lest fetal blood cells entered her circulation during placental bleeding (see Chapter 13).

At 38 weeks, the patient goes to theatre for vaginal examination, with or without general anaesthetic, where the theatre staff are prepared for immediate caesarean section should bleeding occur or placenta praevia of Type II, III or IV be diagnosed. If vaginal examination reveals no abnormality, the membranes are ruptured and labour is allowed to proceed normally.

If bleeding is severe, the patient must be resuscitated and then surgery may be indicated. Once the fetal heartbeat is absent, all hope for the baby's life must be abandoned and the mother's health is of prime importance, with the least trauma by intervention.

6 Disorders of Pregnancy

Disorders associated with pregnancy are considered in four sections in this chapter: minor discomforts, major disorders, diseases associated with pregnancy and chronic diseases occurring during pregnancy.

MINOR DISCOMFORTS OF PREGNANCY

There are many discomforts which occur during pregnancy but there are two main causes:

hormones of pregnancy, and

pressure of the growing uterus.

Minor disorders of pregnancy may seem trivial, but good directive advice can help the patient's discomforts and win her confidence in the midwife or nurse.

Morning sickness

Morning sickness occurs in at least 50% of all pregnancies. The nausea classically occurs in the early morning, but can be during the day and is sometimes accompanied by vomiting. The cause is unknown but could be related to the hormone human chorionic gonadotrophin (HCG), which circulates in high levels up to around the 12th week.

The patient should be encouraged to rise slowly, and is often helped by taking a dry biscuit on waking, followed a little later by a cup of tea. She may feel less nauseated during the day if she eats little and often, because it is thought that the nausea is worse with hunger.

If these measures do not help, an antihistamine such as

Debendox may be prescribed. If vomiting becomes severe, the urine should be tested for ketones, and if present the patient should be admitted to hospital to be rehydrated. The condition should subside by about the 12th week.

Heartburn
Acid stomach contents regurgitate into the oesophagus and cause painful heartburn. This is partly because the cardiac sphincter relaxes under the influence of progesterone, and partly because of pressure from the enlarging uterus.

Small, light meals should be advised and alkaline preparations may be helpful.

Constipation
Constipation is fairly common, especially in late pregnancy, caused by progesterone relaxing smooth muscle of the intestine. It is best treated by extra fluid and dietary adjustment in the form of extra fruit, green vegetables and roughage. If this is inadequate, a mild aperient such as Senokot may be advised.

Frequency of micturition
Frequency of micturition is usually caused by pressure of the uterus on the urinary bladder. This occurs during the first 12 weeks until the uterus rises up out of the pelvis, and again in late pregnancy when the fetal head descends into the pelvis.

Frequency of micturition must be distinguished from urinary infection, and if it is accompanied by pain or a burning sensation a sample of urine should be sent to the laboratory and the appropriate treatment given (see page 82).

Pruritus vulvae
Irritation of the vulva may result from poor hygiene or monilial infection. The urine should be tested because

pruritus vulvae may be associated with glycosuria. Treatment is related to the cause (see Chapter 21).

Vaginal discharge

There is a normal increase in cervical secretions during pregnancy and these pass through the vagina. However, patients are especially susceptible to monilial infection during pregnancy, or there may be other infection. Abnormal discharges and treatment are described in Chapter 22.

The doctor should be informed if there is a bloodstained or offensive discharge.

Varicose veins

Varicose veins may develop or, if already present, worsen during pregnancy. This is caused both by the effect of progesterone and by the pressure of the uterus impeding venous return from the legs. Varicose veins predispose to deep vein thrombosis and care should therefore be taken to improve circulation.

Long periods of standing should be avoided and it may be necessary to wear support tights, elastic stockings or a crepe bandage. These should be put on before rising, to prevent the veins overfilling with blood.

Varicose veins of the vulva are very painful and a vulval pad may give support and ease. These are potentially dangerous as they may rupture during delivery. Haemorrhoids are often troublesome and care should be taken to avoid constipation. Anaesthetic suppositories give some relief.

All types of varicose veins regress after delivery and active treatment is usually avoided for at least six weeks so that a true assessment of the situation can be made.

Cramp

Cramp in the legs is quite common and very painful. It may

be caused by lack of vitamin B, calcium, or possibly by ischaemia of the leg muscles.

Oedema

Oedema of the ankles is not uncommon in pregnancy and may be of no consequence, and the discomfort may be relieved by elevating the legs. However, if oedema is evident elsewhere, it is likely to be of pathological origin and may be a sign of pre-eclampsia.

Backache

Backache occurs partly because of the relaxation of ligaments during pregnancy, and partly because many women adopt poor posture to balance the weight of the fetus. The nurse should correct a patient's bad posture such that the abdomen is pulled in, with the back straight, not hollowed. The patient should be advised to wear stable shoes and take adequate rest. Occasionally a mild analgesic may be necessary.

Insomnia

Sleep is often disturbed in late pregnancy by the discomforts of fetal movements, frequency of micturition and the difficulty in finding a comfortable position. The patient should be advised to take adequate rest, even if she does not sleep, with an afternoon rest. Relaxation exercises may help her.

Insomnia may be a manifestation of some deep-seated anxiety or fear and this must not be overlooked, and expert help obtained if necessary.

MAJOR DISORDERS OF PREGNANCY

Pre-eclampsia

Pre-eclampsia is a serious condition occuring in 10% of all pregnancies, usually after the 28th week. There are many different theories about the cause, but none of them is entirely proven yet.

Dangers The patient may develop eclampsia, renal failure, or have an accidental antepartum haemorrhage, any of which could be fatal. The fetus might die in utero because of changes which take place in the placenta.

Signs There are three cardinal signs: hypertension (blood pressure over 140/90), oedema, and proteinuria. If two of these three are present, then the patient is said to have pre-eclampsia.

Management The aim of management is to prevent complications, that is of eclampsia in the mother and intrauterine anoxia in the fetus.

Complete bed rest improves the circulation to the uterus, thereby improving placental function, and may help to lower the blood pressure. Rest may be improved with the use of sedatives at night and, if the pre-eclampsia is severe, during the day. Obstetricians vary widely in their choice of anti-hypertensive or diuretic drugs.

In addition to ensuring rest (which is not easy when the mother feels perfectly well), the nurse's role is to make observations to monitor the well-being of mother and fetus.

Observations of the mother The maternal blood pressure is recorded at least twice daily, and the mother's urine is tested for proteinuria daily. Fluid intake and urinary output are recorded and oedema is observed both visually and by weighing the patient. Any worsening of the condition, such as vomiting, severe headache, epigastric pain or visual disturbances such as flashing lights must be reported to the doctor immediately because these signs precede eclampsia.

Observations of the fetus Clinical examination is carried out by the midwife or doctor, every day whilst the mother is in hospital, to assess fetal growth and listen to the fetal heart. Special tests will also be carried out, particularly placental function tests, cardiotocographs, and ultrasound scans. These are described in detail in Chapter 4.

The condition usually improves with this treatment, but if it does not, induction of labour will be considered. The risk of eclampsia or intrauterine anoxia (if the pregnancy is allowed to continue) must be balanced against the risk of prematurity (if induction is carried out too early) and this should be explained carefully to the patient and her husband.

Eclampsia

Eclampsia is diagnosed when fits occur and is a very serious condition because of the danger to the patient's life. Maternal death can occur from two factors: the *hypertension* can cause haemorrhage, thrombosis or uraemia, and the *fits* can cause asphyxia and pulmonary oedema with associated pneumonia or cardiac failure. The fetus is at risk from anoxia, and intrauterine death occurs in 40% of cases.

Signs The fits are epileptiform in nature and are preceded by a sharp rise in blood pressure and other signs (see 'Observations of the mother' in 'Pre-eclampsia').

Management The aims of management are to prevent fatal complications, control the fits, and to lower the blood pressure.

First aid is given to prevent death from asphyxia, by clearing the airway and giving oxygen as soon as possible. The patient should never be left alone, and oxygen, suction apparatus and postanaesthetic instruments should remain at the bedside.

Fits are thought to be precipitated by peripheral stimulation, hence the patient is nursed in a quiet, darkened room, with the minimum of disturbance until the fits are controlled. According to the prescription anticonvulsant and hypotensive drugs are administered in various cocktails, such as Heminevrin and Apresoline intravenous infusion.

Labour may start spontaneously or it may be induced. Eclampsia can also occur postpartum.

Hyperemesis gravidarum

Hyperemesis gravidarum, or excessive vomiting, of pregnancy is uncommon but serious. There is a slightly higher incidence with multiple pregnancy.

Signs The morning sickness of early pregnancy persists and becomes more severe, the patient vomiting after meals and sometimes between meals. She begins to show signs of dehydration and ketosis, with a dry skin, sunken eyes, furred tongue, sore lips, and offensive breath. The urine is concentrated and scanty, containing ketones.

Treatment The patient should be admitted to hospital, and given a full medical examination to exclude other conditions which might cause vomiting. A mild sedative such as phenobarbitone 60 mg three times a day and a light diet may be adequate treatment.

If the condition is severe, the blood electrolytes should be investigated, intravenous dextrose infusion given to treat the dehydration and a nasogastric tube inserted and aspirated regularly to alleviate the vomiting. Some obstetricians may order an antiemetic drug.

General skin and mouth care are essential for the patient's comfort. Temperature charts and a fluid balance chart should be maintained, and the urine tested for ketones at regular intervals.

Once the general condition improves, oral feeding can be resumed. The cause of hyperemesis gravidarum is not known, but in many cases there is some underlying emotional factor.

Retroverted incarcerated uterus

Occasionally in patients with congenital retroversion, the uterus becomes incarcerated. Treatment is first of all to relieve retention of urine by continuous bladder drainage. The patient should rest in bed and lie prone for as long as possible, which encourages the uterus to fall foward out of the pelvis. Within a few days the uterus is palpable in the abdomen and there is no further retention.

DISEASES ASSOCIATED WITH PREGNANCY

Anaemia

Anaemia is diagnosed when the haemoglobin (Hb) falls below 10.4 g per ml. This is a relative anaemia because haemodilution normally occurs during pregnancy. It is treated because there could be serious consequences if blood loss at delivery were above average, and because it makes the patient feel debilitated, tired and listless.

There are different types of anaemia seen in pregnancy.

Iron deficiency anaemia is caused by the insufficient intake of iron and by the high demand for iron, especially in multiple pregnancy or grande multiparity.

Management is often by prophylaxis using oral compounds such as Ferrograd Folic. If anaemia is diagnosed, ferrous sulphate may be prescribed. Once the Hb falls below 9 g, a total dose infusion of iron-dextran (Imferon) may be given intravenously, or near the time of delivery packed red cells may be transfused.

Megaloblastic anaemia in pregnancy is caused by folic

acid deficiency. This occurs in the latter half of pregnancy and is treated with folic acid 15 mg daily.

Sickle cell anaemia occurs in West Indians or Negro blood, and **thalassaemia** occurs in Mediterranean people. Both are haemolytic anaemias and blood transfusions may become necessary.

Cystitis

Cystitis is inflammation of the urinary bladder; the causative organism is usually *Escherichia coli*.

Signs and symptoms The patient feels vaguely unwell, with low abdominal pain, frequency and a burning pain on micturition. The urine is opalescent, acid in reaction and has an offensive fishy odour. Bacteriological examination detects pus cells, red cells, and organisms.

Treatment The patient is encouraged to drink large amounts of fluids, at least 3 litres daily. Potassium citrate and hyoscyamus is given to render the urine alkaline and to ease the dysuria. Sulphonamides or nitrofurantoin may be prescribed.

Asymptomatic bacteriuria is not uncommon during pregnancy which, if untreated, can rapidly ascend to the kidney, causing pyelonephritis.

Pyelonephritis

Pyelonephritis is a bacterial infection involving the ureter, renal pelvis and kidney. The most common organism involved is *Escherichia coli*.

Signs and symptoms The onset is often sudden, with pain radiating from the loin to the groin. High temperature accompanied by rigors may occur. Repeated vomiting, anorexia and general malaise are usually present. The urine may appear opalescent, is usually acid in reaction and has a characteristic fishy odour.

Treatment The patient should be kept in bed to rest until the fever subsides, and she should be encouraged to drink large quantities of fluid. She should be reassured that the fetus is safe, because she will be very anxious in case she should miscarry.

A clean specimen of urine should be sent for bacteriological examination and the appropriate antibiotic administered. Treatment should be continued for at least three weeks and further specimens of urine should be sent to the laboratory.

Pyelonephritis may recur postnatally and all patients should be reassessed four months after delivery, and appropriate treatment given if required.

Deep vein thrombosis

There is a slightly increased risk of deep vein thrombosis during pregnancy because high levels of circulating oestrogen increase blood coagulability and because venous return is impeded by the pressure of the growing uterus. An early diagnosis should be made by examining the patient's legs regularly, and treatment is instituted with rest and support to the leg.

CHRONIC DISEASES IN PREGNANCY

Cardiac conditions

Cardiac conditions tend to become worse during pregnancy because the work load on the heart increases. The worsening of symptoms is most easily explained using the grades of cardiac involvement, so, for example, a woman with Grade I involvement (no symptoms) is likely to pass to Grade II (symptoms on exertion), or from Grade III (symptoms with any activity) to Grade IV (symptoms at rest).

Prolonged admission to hospital may be necessary during the antenatal period. Labour will be kept short and sedation given to prevent maternal distress—an epidural anaesthetic is ideal. Oxytocic drugs are used with extreme caution in third stage, because the resultant sudden strong uterine contractions might force 500 ml of blood from the uterine circulation into the general circulation, with such force as to precipitate congestive cardiac failure.

Prophylactic antibiotics are usually prescribed to prevent subacute bacterial endocarditis. Postnatal care is likely to be extended in order to give the patient extra rest.

Diabetes mellitus

Diabetes during pregnancy can cause several complications, in both mother and baby, unless it is well controlled. The diabetes and the pregnancy each affect one another.

Dangers Pregnancy worsens diabetes because the need for insulin increases, but it fluctuates widely causing instability. Diabetic lesions such as retinopathy tend to worsen.

Diabetes complicates pregnancy: there is a higher incidence of pre-eclampsia and polyhydramnios. The fetus is often large (5 kg) which may make vaginal delivery impossible. Intrauterine fetal death is more common after 36 weeks gestation.

Management A known diabetic is seen more frequently, at least once every fortnight, in order to assess her condition and readjust insulin dosage. Any patient with suspected or potential diabetes should have a glucose tolerance test, so that treatment can be instituted before complications arise.

Glycosuria often occurs in normal pregnancy, therefore blood glucose measurements are of more value than urine samples in diabetes. Recent research has shown satisfactory control of diabetes by self-monitoring of blood glucose at home, using a Reflomat machine. The patient charts blood glucose results several times per day, once per fortnight, to give a comprehensive profile of blood glucose levels. If this is impossible, the patient must be admitted to hospital for stabilization, especially if she is uncooperative with self-management.

Patients who were already diabetic are accustomed to looking after themselves, administering insulin. This independence need not be removed during pregnancy: indeed, most patients are happy to help in their special care, knowing that this will make the baby healthier.

Labour may be induced early, but the risk of intrauterine death must be weighed against the risk of death from prematurity.

Postpartum, maternal insulin requirements return to the non-pregnant state immediately. The baby should be observed closely or, if necessary, given specific treatment.

Essential hypertension

Essential hypertension, or hypertension associated with renal disease, may be present in a pregnant woman. The blood pressure is raised before pre-eclampsia normally arises, although if a patient is late seeking antenatal care, essential hypertension is difficult to distinguish from pre-eclampsia.

The patient has an increased risk of pre-eclampsia, haemorrhage from placental abruption, or cerebrovascular accident. The life of the fetus is at risk from chronic intrauterine anoxia because of poor placental function.

Management The patient's blood pressure is monitored carefully during pregnancy. She may be admitted to hospital for extra rest, and hypotensive drugs are sometimes used but this carries risk to the fetus. Early induction of labour is usually indicated when placental function tests are poor, to prevent intrauterine fetal death. When hypertension is very severe, termination of pregnancy must be considered.

Tuberculosis

Tuberculosis has little effect on pregnancy and with modern treatment pregnancy has no adverse effect on the disease, although the mother is likely to be anaemic. Special therapy is continued throughout the pregnancy.

After delivery, the baby is protected by an inoculation with BCG, but he should be isolated from the mother until this has taken effect (about six weeks) unless isonized resistant BCG is given, when the baby can be nursed by his mother.

All babies are given BCG if the mother (or relatives) has had positive sputum within the previous two years.

7 Physiology and Management of Labour

THE PELVIS

The structure and shape of the pelvis are important in obstetrics because it is a fixed structure through which the fetus must pass on its way from the uterus to the vagina. The pelvis can either assist or inhibit the descent of the fetus during labour.

The regions of the pelvis

The pelvis is described as having two regions, named according to their significance in obstetrics.

The false pelvis The false pelvis is so called because it is of little significance during labour. It lies above the pelvic brim and is formed by the wings of the ilium.

The true pelvis The true pelvis is a bony basin and is significant because it forms the canal through which the fetus travels. It has three main areas: the inlet brim, the cavity, and the outlet.

Inlet pelvic brim In the normal female gynaecoid pelvis, the inlet pelvic brim is oval in shape, which naturally encourages the fetal head to enter sideways. Once the biparietal diameter has passed through the brim, the head is said to have engaged. If the pelvis is very narrow and

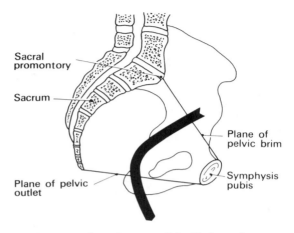

Fig. 7.1 Diagram to show the curve of the birth canal.

engagement does not occur, problems are likely during labour because there will be cephalopelvic disproportion (page 113).

The pelvic brim is bounded by the promontory and wings (ala) of the sacrum posteriorly, the iliopectineal line laterally and the upper borders of the pubic rami and pubic symphysis anteriorly.

The cavity of the pelvis The cavity is the circular space between the brim above and the outlet below. Its borders make the birth canal curved because the curved sacrum posteriorly is about 7 cm longer than the symphysis pubis anteriorly (Fig. 7.1).

The outlet of the pelvis The obstetric outlet, though not anatomically the lowest border of the pelvis, is the final bony structure through which the fetus has to pass, and is important because the size and angles of the bones can either facilitate delivery or cause obstruction to the fetus.

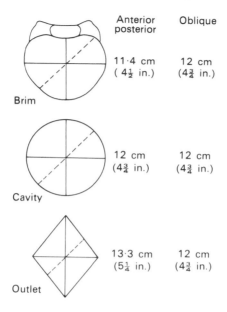

	Anterior posterior	Oblique
Brim	11·4 cm (4½ in.)	12 cm (4¾ in.)
Cavity	12 cm (4¾ in.)	12 cm (4¾ in.)
Outlet	13·3 cm (5¼ in.)	12 cm (4¾ in.)

Fig. 7.2 Diagram showing shape and approximate dimensions of a normal female pelvis.

The obstetric outlet forms a diamond shape bounded by the pubic arch, the ischial spines, sacrospinous ligaments and lower border of the sacrum. (The coccyx is pulled back during labour.)

Dimensions An assessment of the pelvis is made during pregnancy in order to anticipate any disproportion and prevent any trauma to either mother or baby. It can be seen (Fig. 7.2) that the widest (transverse) diameter at the brim becomes the narrowest (anteroposterior) diameter at the outlet—this encourages rotation of the fetus during labour.

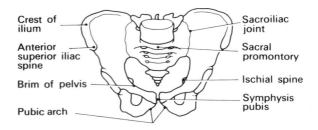

Fig. 7.3 The female pelvis.

Structure

The pelvis consists of two innominate bones, one sacrum and one coccyx (Fig. 7.3).

Innominate bone Each innominate bone is the result of fusion of three bones, the ilium, ischium and pubes, which form the anterior and lateral parts of the pelvis.

Ilium The ilium is the upper expanded portion which provides on its posterior surface attachment for the gluteal muscles (see Fig. 26.1). The upper border, easily felt exteriorly in all but the very obese, is called the iliac crest, with sharp anterior and posterior prominences called spines. The concave anterior surface is called the iliac fossa. A ridge on its inner aspect is known as the iliopectineal line.

Ischium The ischium is the lower part of the innominate bone. It has a large tuberosity and its internal aspect forms the side walls of the true pelvis. Protruding inwards from its posterior edge, about 5 cm above the tuberosity, is a projection known as the ischial spine. This is a feature felt on vaginal examination and is one of the important landmarks in pregnancy (see 'The outlet of the pelvis'). The spine separates the greater and the lesser sciatic notch.

Pubis The pubic bone, or front portion of the innominate bone, has a square-shaped body and two projections, or rami. These rami, together with those of the ischium, enclose the obturator foramen. The pubic rami form the pubic arch which in a gynaecoid-type pelvis is an angle of 90°. It is important to estimate this angle because a narrow arch impedes the exit of the fetus.

The sacrum The sacrum, together with the coccyx, forms the back of the pelvis. It is a wedge-shaped bone consisting of five fused vertebrae and perforated by four sets of foramena through which pass the sacral nerves. Its inner aspect is concave and forms what is known as the hollow of the sacrum. The first sacral vertebra overhangs the sacral hollow and the central point is known as the sacral promontory: the distance between this and the pubic bones is important in obstetrics (see 'The inlet of the pelvis').

The coccyx The coccyx is formed from four rudimentary vertebrae fused together, and is capable of a little movement in pregnancy.

Pelvic joints There are three pelvic joints: the *sacroiliac* joint, the *symphysis pubis* and the *sacrococcygeal* joint (see Fig. 7.3). The range of movements in these joints is increased during pregnancy because the hormones cause softening in the retaining ligaments. This gives rise to the characteristic rolling gait of pregnant women but can occasionally cause joint pain during the last trimester.

Pelvic ligaments There are a number of pelvic ligaments but the two of special significance are the *sacrospinous*, passing from sacrum to coccyx across to the ischial spine, and the *sacrotuberous* ligament passing from sacrum to the ischial tuberosity.

LABOUR

Pregnancy is normally brought to its end at around 40 weeks gestation. What causes the onset of labour is not known but it is heralded by several signs.

1. The commencement of regular, perceptible uterine contractions that can be felt by the patient and elicited by the observer.

2. A 'show', this is the extrusion of the operculum from the cervical canal. The patient notices thick, bloodstained mucus which passes *per vaginam*.

3. Rupture of the membranes: this may be an early or late sign.

Normal labour is said to occur when the mother, by her own efforts, delivers a live healthy baby by a vertex presentation. The duration of labour is variable but should be completed within 24 hours. Primiparous patients tend to have a longer labour than multigravidae.

Labour divides into three stages.

First stage from the onset of uterine contractions until full dilatation of the cervix.

Second stage from full dilatation of the cervix to complete expulsion of the baby.

Third stage from the birth of the baby to the complete expulsion of the placenta and membranes.

THE FIRST STAGE OF LABOUR

Physiology

The purpose of labour is to expel the fetus from the uterus and to do this it must open up the passageway and provide a propelling force. Two problems have to be overcome, first to provide sufficient force without fatiguing the uterus, and second to maintain an adequate oxygen supply to the fetus.

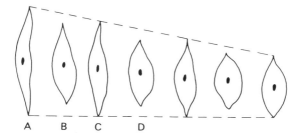

Fig. 7.4 Diagram to illustrate retraction. Uterine muscle fibre: A relaxed; B contracted; C relaxed but with retraction; D contracted but shorter and thicker than B.

When the uterus contracts its blood supply is diminished and the placenta is squeezed, this reduces the oxygen flow to the fetus so it is necessary to have a compensation period of relaxation. This being the case, there would never be enough force to propel the fetus down the birth canal, so another factor enters into uterine activity called *retraction*. When the muscle fibres of the uterus contract, they also retract, that is, by internal molecular rearrangement they become permanently shorter, but they do relax. Thus over a period of time the length of the uterus is decreased and the walls become thicker (Fig. 7.4).

In labour the upper uterine segment is the active area of the uterus and it becomes smaller and thicker. This exerts a pull on the less active lower uterine segment, the maximum pull being directed to the weakest point—that is, the opening or external os. This is gradually pulled upwards until the cervical canal is obliterated, a process known as 'taking up' of the cervix or effacement. The continued upward pull now dilates the cervix, i.e. enlarges the opening (Fig. 7.5). In parous patients, effacement and dilatation usually occur simultaneously.

During this time the fetus is being forced downwards by the

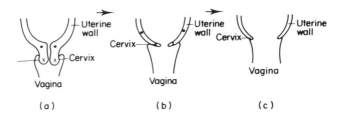

Fig. 7.5 Diagram to show effacement and dilatation of the cervix.

force of contractions against this resistance. If the membranes are intact, some liquor amnii is trapped between the head and the membranes: this is called the forewaters. These help in cervical dilatation and usually rupture near the end of the first stage of labour.

When the dilatation is sufficient to allow the head to pass through, this is called full dilatation of the cervix and its diameter usually measures 10 cm.

Management of first stage

Assessment of needs The patient's physical condition and stage in labour are assessed either in hospital or at home if a home confinement is planned. The earlier the patient is seen in labour, the more unhurried and relaxed can be the assessment of her needs. Indeed, the actual assessment can be a time when an initial rapport is established with the patient. This not only helps a patient psychologically but also physiologically, because when muscles are relaxed the cervix dilates more quickly.

History Examination of the patient consists of reviewing her history followed by a physical examination. Any details taken at antenatal visits are checked from her 'cooperation card' or medical case notes, because some aspects of her history are relevant to labour and its management (see Chapter 4). Her present history is recorded so that the stage of labour may be assessed both now and subsequently. Particular attention is paid to signs of labour described on page 92.

Physical examination The patient is examined to check her physical health. Blood pressure, urinalysis and signs of oedema are observed because these give signs of pre-eclampsia. The temperature is taken because pyrexia must be treated, especially if it indicates infected liquor. The maternal pulse rate is recorded because tachycardia could be a sign of maternal ketoacidosis or other disorder. The abdomen is examined to find the position, presentation and lie of the fetus, the fetal heart listened to and the strength and frequency of the contractions noted. A vaginal or rectal examination may be carried out to assess the degree of dilatation of the cervix and confirm the position of the baby.

Written records All of these findings must be recorded accurately, in order to provide continuity of care between staff and to demonstrate clearly the progress in labour so that management can be re-evaluated according to this vital information. These written records are documents which can be used in a court of law for up to 21 years after birth, as evidence of care or negligence.

Planning care In a normal labour, most mothers appreciate taking an active part in 'giving birth' rather than passively 'being delivered'. There is no need for professionals to dictate what the mother does without discussion or explanation, even when there is some abnormality which calls for active intervention.

When planning care, the nurse can often take her cue from the mother, whose desires are protected by a natural instinct for survival and comfort. However, the nurse should use her position as non-participant in order to bring calm, serene reassurance which a mother herself cannot always maintain when she is so painfully involved.

This serenity can be brought about in different ways, according to the patient's individual need. She may appreciate having the lumbar area rubbed or stroked firmly; she almost always benefits from a quiet, controlled voice when being addressed; she may wish for stark lights to be dimmed whenever their glare is unnecessary; she may want to adopt the position of maximum comfort even if that is not in bed. When a mother does not know what she wants, the nurse must win her confidence and give firm suggestions and guidance.

Giving care Normal labour inevitably progresses of its own accord: indeed, the fact that labour is so inescapable daunts many mothers. The nurse's role is to encourage the patient using whatever means the patient expressed as her wish during discussions and planning of care. Observations must be carried out in order to detect early signs of deviation from normal and prevent severe complications.

Observations of the mother are continued (see 'Physical examination', page 95). Fetal wellbeing is observed by listening to the fetal heart via a Pinard's stethoscope, or by continuous monitoring (see Chapter 4 and Fig. 4.10.) The liquor is observed because meconium staining is a sign of fetal distress. These observations are important because the fetus is at risk during labour, especially from intrauterine anoxia.

Maintenance of hygiene is important so that the patient feels fresh. Simple steps such as wiping her face with a cool sponge, brushing the teeth and combing her hair, all help towards boosting her morale.

The perineal area is sometimes shaved, although the value

of doing so is questionable since shaving does not reduce infection from a laceration or episiotomy. If the rectum is full, suppositories or even an enema may be given, after which the patient usually enjoys a warm bath or shower.

Throughout the first stage of labour the patient is encouraged to pass urine every two hours, because a full bladder may cause a diminution of uterine contractions. As the bladder is pulled up into the abdominal cavity the urethra is stretched and sensation is less, therefore the patient feels no urge to empty her bladder. This sensation is completely reduced when epidural anaesthetic is used, so the nurse must remember to offer bedpans.

As labour progresses, solid food and milky drinks should be avoided because the stomach empties slowly in time of stress, and if an anaesthetic becomes necessary there would be a danger of inhalation of vomit. In a normal labour, the patient may drink as much water as she desires, which helps to prevent dehydration. Intravenous fluids are occasionally indicated to treat ketoacidosis, and are always given when the patient has an epidural anaesthetic because of the danger of rapid fall of blood pressure.

The patient may adopt the position most comfortable to her during labour. If she is in hospital she may prefer to sit in the day room than be confined to bed or, if she is at home, she may continue with light tasks which distract her from the contractions. She should not be allowed to lie prone, because this causes the heavy uterus to impede blood flow via the inferior vena cava.

The husband has an important role to play if he can stay with his wife, by holding her hand and gently rubbing her back during contractions. If he cannot be there, the nurse should be as available as possible to sit with her. Patients often feel neglected; almost all patients are fearful of being left alone in labour, so when the nurse must go away for a short time she should explain how she can be called back promptly. Even if the nurse has recorded observations every 15 minutes, this often seems inadequate to a patient unless she gives extra care by a few words and a little encouragement every time.

Pain relief When contractions start, the pain starts in the hollow of the sacrum and works round to the abdomen, rather like dysmenorrhoea but becoming progressively more severe. Eventually most patients will require something to help them to cope: they may be helped by psychoprophylaxis (Chapter 4), or analgesics may be given by injection, inhalation or locally such as via an epidural cannula.

If the patient has learned a method of psychoprophylaxis, such as at National Childbirth Trust Classes, the nurse should help the patient to continue with the exercises by reinforcing any teaching during each contraction.

Intramuscular injection of pethidine hydrochloride 100 to

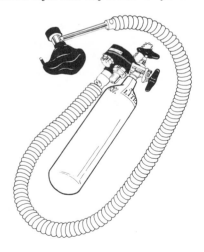

Fig. 7.6 The Entonox inhaler.

150 mg is frequently recommended. Oral pethidine is not given in labour because of the likelihood of vomiting.

Inhalation analgesia such as nitrous oxide and oxygen may be given via an Entonox machine (Fig. 7.6), or methoxyflurane (Penthrane) in a Cardiff inhaler, or trichloroethylene in a Tecota (Fig. 7.7) or Emotril inhaler. The patient administers

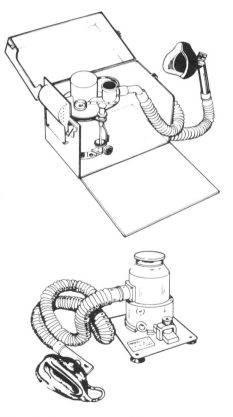

Fig. 7.7 Trichloroethylene apparatus. Above: Tecota inhaler. Below: Emotril inhaler.

this herself, but if she has not become familiar with the apparatus at parentcraft classes, the nurse must help her.

Local anaesthetic can be inserted into the epidural space, giving complete freedom from sensory stimuli below the waist. This anaesthetic is even sufficient to allow caesarean section to be painless. Spinal anaesthetic has a less comprehensive effect. Blocking the pudendal nerves (paracervical nerve block) may be carried out in the second stage of labour.

As the patient nears the end of the first stage of labour she feels she cannot stand much more, and may become very distressed. She should be reassured with the information that this is a normal and encouraging sign that she is approaching the second stage of labour.

THE SECOND STAGE OF LABOUR

The second stage of labour is the stage of expulsion of the fetus. The cervix has dilated sufficiently to allow the fetus to pass through, and as contraction and retraction occur the fetus is thrust down the birth canal (Fig. 7.8). The fetus is expelled following a curve (see Fig. 7.1). The patient often emits a grunting sound as she pushes down involuntarily because the abdominal muscles and diaphragm assist the expulsive forces which she cannot resist.

Management

Throughout the second and third stage, the patient must not be left alone and she should be moved to the room where delivery is to take place and where any equipment is ready.

Observations of the fetal heartbeat and maternal pulse, and frequency and strength of contractions are continued every few minutes to detect the earliest signs of distress. The vulval area is inspected during a contraction and it will be noticed that as the presenting part descends the anus dilates, the perineum bulges forward and finally the labia gape.

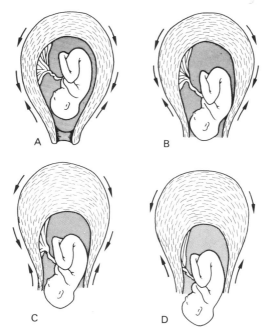

Fig. 7.8 **Expulsion of the fetus from the uterus. A shows bag of membranes intact. B, C and D show bag of membranes ruptured. The arrows indicate muscular contraction which contract the fundus and dilate the cervix.**

If the bladder is thought to be full, the patient is unlikely to be able to pass urine and a catheter should be passed. Catheterization is more difficult because of the proximity of the urethra to the distended vagina and because, as the bladder is pulled into the abdominal cavity, the urethra lengthens to 15 or 16 cm (normally 3 cm in length).

The position of the patient is decided to suit the comfort of the mother and the midwife and to allow muscles to assist the passage of the baby. She may sit semirecumbent with her knees flexed, or she may lie in the left lateral position and raise one leg as the baby is born, or she may prefer to squat with or without the support of a birth stool (Fig. 7.9).

Despite the climatic intensity of contractions, the patient is usually thrilled to know that she will soon see her baby. Inhalation analgesia is sometimes continued but most patients prefer to be free to concentrate on bearing down. Continual encouragement is vital to the patient.

When delivery is imminent, the midwife or doctor dons sterile gown and gloves; the vulval and perineal areas are cleansed with an antiseptic solution such as Hibitane 1 in 1000, and the surrounding areas covered with sterile towels. As the head emerges, it is kept flexed in order to control its exit and prevent undue damage to the perineum. When the widest diameter distends the vulva (crowning), the patient is asked to pant so as to prevent her pushing and to allow the remainder of the head and face to be born slowly.

There is usually a pause between contractions at this point, and the mother may be excited to see her baby's head. Meanwhile the midwife feels for the umbilical cord around the baby's neck by sliding a finger under the pubic arch, and if present it should be slipped over the head or clamped with two arterial pressure forceps and cut between them. This is to prevent undue tightening around the baby's neck when the body is subsequently delivered. If time permits before the next contraction, the eyes are swabbed and the nose and mouth wiped with gauze to remove mucus.

The next contraction completes the delivery of shoulders and body in an upward direction, and still following the physiological curve (see Fig. 7.1), the baby can either be placed directly on to the mother's abdomen or be given straight into her waiting arms. This is the moment of supreme joy for both parents, when they hear the baby grasp and cry and see his tiny features. Their two questions are always, *'Is he alright?'* and *'Is it a girl or boy?'*. To new parents, the

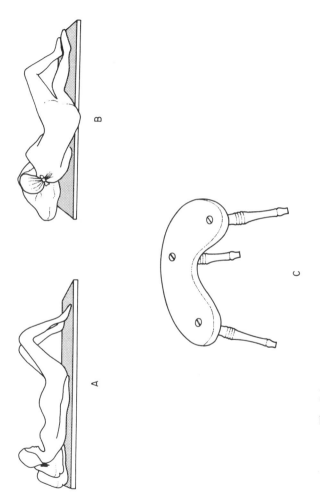

Fig. 7.9 Positions for delivery. A: Dorsal position; B: Left lateral position; C: A birth stool.

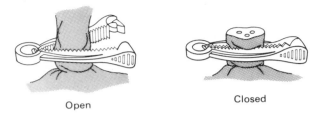

Open   Closed

Fig. 7.10 Cord clamp (open and closed).

most minor problem which takes the baby away unexpectedly, even for a few minutes, seems disastrous; therefore if there are any immediate problems which require treatment, such as asphyxia, they should always be given explanations.

The cord is now tied or clamped (Fig. 7.10), and cut. The air passages can normally be cleared by the use of a mucus extractor (Fig. 7.11). If the delivery is in hospital, an identity

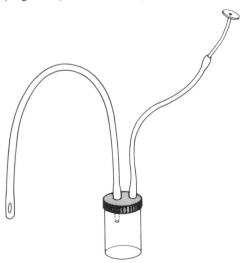

Fig. 7.11 Mucus extractor.

label bearing the patient's name and the sex of the baby is put on to the baby's wrist or ankle, in the presence of the mother.

The baby loses body heat very quickly, therefore he is dried immediately and kept warm by close contact in the mother's arms, covered with a sterile towel (see Fig. 7.12). If this is impossible, he should be wrapped warmly in blankets and placed in a warm cot. However, it is thought that skin-to-skin contact not only keeps the baby warm, but also enhances bonding at this important early stage, and that early breast-feeding which often follows quite naturally tends to form a pattern for good breast-feeding throughout babyhood.

THE THIRD STAGE OF LABOUR

Even after the baby is safely born, labour is incomplete and the third stage is hazardous for the mother, with the possibility of haemorrhage. Bleeding is normally controlled by retracted muscle fibres which squeeze the blood vessels and prevent bleeding. As the baby is born the uterus retracts markedly, the placental site becomes much smaller but the placenta, being inelastic, buckles and becomes stripped from the uterine wall (Fig. 7.14). Bleeding occurs and a clot forms behind the placenta, the retroplacental clot, which further helps to shear the placenta off the uterine wall, and its own weight carries it down into the vagina. The patient is not usually aware of this.

Management

In order to assist nature and reduce haemorrhage, ergometrine maleate 0.5 mg or Syntometrine 1 ml (containing oxytocin 5 units and ergometrine maleate 0.25 mg) may have been given intramuscularly when the head crowned or when the anterior shoulder was delivered, according to preference.

Once the baby is born, a receiver is laid close to the vulva to catch the liquor and blood which may escape from the

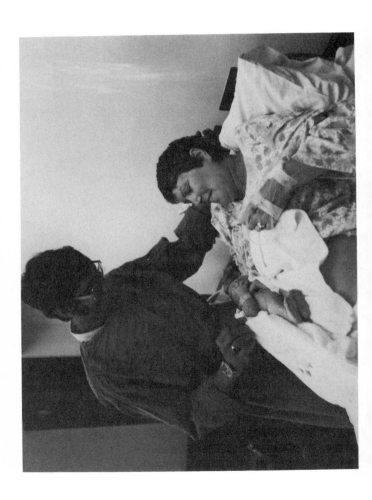

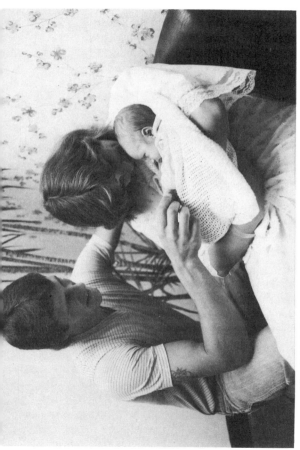

Figs. 7.12 & 7.13 Whether the delivery was at home or in hospital, the baby and the parents take the first opportunity to begin to get to know each other; by looking, by listening, by 'talking', and by touching.

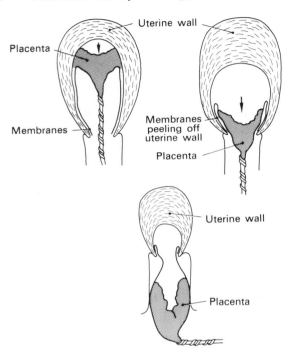

Fig. 7.14 Diagrams showing the placenta being expelled within the bag of membranes.

vagina. A dry sheet should be pulled beneath her buttocks and a warm covering placed over her chest. The mother can easily become chilled after her exertions of pushing, therefore she should not be left exposed for any longer than necessary.

The method of delivery of the placenta varies. Each method is a skilful procedure which must be learnt at the bedside so that the manoeuvres can be carried out at the correct time. The uterus must be in a state of contraction, otherwise inversion (turning inside out) of the uterus might occur. The cord may be grasped and the placenta pulled out by controlled cord traction, or the mother may bear down gently, and deliver it by maternal effort. Pressure on the fundus, using the uterus as a piston, tends to damage the uterine supports.

When delivery is completed, the vulva and perineum are swabbed and inspected for lacerations, a vulval pad is placed in position and the patient left to rest in a dry bed. The placenta and membranes are inspected to make sure nothing has been retained, and the blood loss is measured.

The midwife must record in the patient's notes details of the delivery, lacerations and blood loss, together with the sex and condition of the baby, and its weight when available. She is required to notify the birth within 36 hours to the District Health Authority in the area in which the baby was born. This is not the same as the registration of birth made by the parents within 42 days of birth.

First aid at a delivery

The nurse is often anxious in case her assistance should be sought when a woman suddenly delivers in a public place or in a nearby house. There is little she can do, in that the baby will deliver itself without assistance, and therefore she should give attention to a few priorities.

The aims in first aid are to bring an air of calm (however unconfident she herself may feel) so as to make the delivery seem less of a panic which can be traumatic to both mother and baby; to clear the baby's airways and to keep him as warm as possible.

Calm can be restored by removing unnecessary people and helping the mother into a comfortable position. She may lie down or sit supported, with cumbersome clothing removed. The time of delivery should be noted.

The baby's air passages should be cleared and eyes wiped using a clean handkerchief. He should be wrapped in something warm and held closely by the mother, or placed between her legs if the cord is short. The cord should **not** be cut.

The placenta may slide out of the vagina, in which case it should be wrapped up and left beside the baby. If bleeding occurs the nurse may lay her hand on the abdomen just above the umbilicus to try to identify the uterus and massage it until it becomes firm: bleeding should then cease. On no other occasion should the abdomen be touched, as this might cause bleeding. The nurse should stay with mother and baby until the ambulance and midwife or doctor arrives.

LACERATIONS OF THE GENITAL TRACT

Lacerations occur when the vaginal outlet is unable to stretch sufficiently to accommodate a large baby. They cause a great deal of discomfort which requires understanding from the nurse. They tend to be less painful than episiotomies, but mild analgesics relieve the pain.

Lacerations can be the site of haemorrhage and third degree lacerations are serious as involvement of the anal sphincter could lead to faecal incontinence.

Lacerations of the perineum are divided into three categories according to the structures involved (see Fig. 21.1).

First degree laceration—involving the skin of the fourchette.
Second degree laceration (and episiotomy, Chapter 8)— involving the skin of the fourchette, the perineum and perineal body.
Third degree laceration—involving the skin of the fourchette, the perineum, perineal body and anal sphincter.

Lacerations are repaired with catgut sutures and occasionally nylon for the skin sutures. Nursing care is described in Chapter 9.

Labial lacerations

Lacerations of the labia are very superficial but, like skin grazes, are rather painful, and analgesics are given for the discomfort. They are not usually severe enough to require suturing, but are kept clean and dry.

Vaginal and cervical lacerations

The cervix is so vascular that a laceration can cause haemorrhage. Both cervical and vaginal lacerations should be sutured.

8 Disorders of Labour

In any apparently normal labour, complications can arise. The most important of these are mentioned in this chapter.

Fetal distress

Fetal distress occurs when the fetus lacks oxygen. The causes are numerous but the signs always the same: the fetal heart rate rises, then becomes slow and irregular and may finally stop. If the membranes have ruptured, there may be evidence of meconium staining (the liquor is greenish in colour) because as the fetus becomes atonic the anal sphincter relaxes and meconium is passed.

Fetal distress must be treated promptly, therefore the nurse's role of observing and then reporting signs is very important. Treatment depends on the cause, and it is usually necessary to delivery the baby as soon as possible.

Maternal distress

Maternal distress is said to occur when the mother feels completely unable to continue in labour. Her exhaustion may be physiological, but it is usually compounded by psychological factors such as being disheartened by the pain or the length of labour. The nurse can help by helping her to understand what is going on and by encouraging her with explanations of her progress. The patient may also require analgesics to relieve the pain and allow her to rest, and an intravenous infusion of dextrose saline. Her condition must be reassessed frequently because labour may need to be terminated by forceps delivery or caesarean section.

Multiple pregnancy

The risk of complications increases in multiple pregnancy and, for this reason, delivery in hospital is recommended. The babies tend to be small; malpresentation of the second fetus is very common (such as breech); and the risk of postpartum haemorrhage is high because of the large placental site.

In the United Kingdom, 1 in 80 pregnancies produces twins, and 1 in 7000 produces triplets.

Prolapse of the cord

Prolapse of the cord occurs when the membranes rupture and, as the liquor gushes out, the cord is swept down past the presenting part. The cord becomes compressed between the fetal head and the maternal pelvis, constituting a serious emergency because the fetus will die from asphyxia unless delivered quickly. If the cervix is fully dilated, forceps can be applied, but more usually this occurs in the first stage of labour and an immediate caesarean section is required.

Prolonged labour

Labour may be prolonged for several reasons.

Cephalopelvic disproportion Sometimes the maternal pelvis is too small to allow the passage of the fetal head, which is known as cephalopelvic disproportion. It is recognized by the failure of the fetal head to enter the pelvis. Minor degrees may be overcome by moulding, otherwise caesarean section is indicated.

Malpresentation and malposition If the fetus does not present by the head, there is malpresentation—that is, a breech, shoulder, face, brow or chin presentation. Malposition occurs when the presentation is cephalic but the occiput is posterior in the pelvis. All these are likely to prolong labour.

Uterine inertia Uterine contractions may be ineffective, they may be poor and infrequent or painful colicky-type contractions which achieve very little. Oxytocin (Syntocinon) may be given intravenously if there are no complicating factors, otherwise caesarean section may be necessary.

Rigid perineum The second stage of labour may be prolonged if the soft parts, particularly the perineum, are rigid and this will slow delivery. The treatment is an episiotomy (see page 118).

Postpartum haemorrhage

Bleeding normally occurs after delivery, but when this exceeds 500 ml it is termed postpartum haemorrhage. This is often preceded by a prolonged labour, and may occur during or after the third stage of labour.

An oxytocic drug such as ergometrine maleate 0.5 mg should be given intravenously or intramuscularly, and the placenta delivered if it is still in the uterus. The pulse, blood pressure and vaginal loss should be recorded until the patient's condition is satisfactory. Resuscitative measures such as blood transfusion may be necessary. Unfortunately, there is still a risk of maternal death from sudden haemorrhage.

OBSTETRIC PROCEDURES ASSOCIATED WITH PREGNANCY AND LABOUR

Insertion of a Shirodkar suture

Patients who have had repeated spontaneous abortions caused by cervical incompetence (a laxity of the cervix), may have a suture inserted in the cervix. This holds the cervix closed, being rather like the purse-string suture done in an appendicetomy (Fig. 8.1). The suture is removed just before term, or earlier if labour commences.

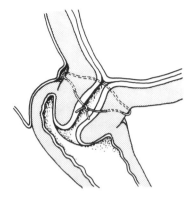

Fig. 8.1 Shirodkar suture.

Ultrasonography

Ultrasonic waves are sound waves above the frequency appreciated by the human ear, over 20 000 cycles/second. These waves are formed into a beam and directed on to the abdomen. When the waves cross a boundary (interface) between two tissues of differing properties, they are reflected back and can be observed on a screen. Ultrasound does not harm the fetus and it may be used with safety in the early weeks of pregnancy. Ultrasound can help in the diagnosis of multiple pregnancy, hydatidiform mole and fetal abnormality. It can locate the placenta and confirm the diagnosis of placenta praevia. Ultrasound can be interpreted to allow accurate measurement of the biparietal diameter which can confirm maturity of the fetus. Repeated scans can show whether fetal growth is occurring normally.

The patient should be warned that she must have a full bladder for ultrasonography.

External cephalic version

Version is a means of altering the presentation of the fetus in

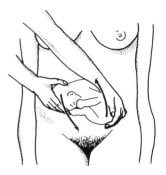

Fig. 8.2 External cephalic version.

utero, the most common being the external cephalic version
(Fig. 8.2). This is performed between the 32nd and 34th
week to turn a breech presentation to a cephalic one.

   This simple manoeuvre can be achieved during an abdominal palpation and is most usually done in the antenatal
clinic. The patient needs to be relaxed and the doctor gently
pushes the baby's head towards its feet until the head lies
over the pelvic brim. If the patient is Rhesus negative, a blood
sample should be taken for a Kleihauer's test (see 'Rhesus
iso-immunization', Chapter 13).

Amnioscopy

Amnionoscopy means viewing the liquor through a special
speculum passed vaginally. If the liquor is golden, it suggests
Rhesus incompatibility (see Chapter 13); and if greenish, it
suggests that meconium is present and the fetus may be
distressed. The same technique may be utilized to take a
specimen of liquor amnii for examination, and also for fetal
blood sampling (page 118).

Induction of labour

Labour may be induced by medical or surgical means. In primigravidae, medical and surgical methods are often combined, but in multiparous patients surgical induction alone is usually sufficient to make labour begin.

Medical induction This normally involves the use of synthetic hormones, administered orally, locally or intravenously. Prostaglandins can be given by oral tablet or by vaginal pessary or gel, to ripen the cervix. Oxytocin (Syntocinon) is given by continuous intravenous infusion. In both cases, the patient's condition must be observed closely, especially uterine activity, because excessive amounts of hormone cause tonic contraction of the uterus.

Some women attempt to induce labour by taking purgatives such as castor oil and hot baths, but their effectiveness is doubtful.

Surgical induction (artificial rupture of the membranes) This is achieved by rupturing the membranes by means of a toothed forcep such as Kocher's, or a Drew Smythe cannula, introduced via the cervix. Liquor amnii drains away; if it gushes out there is a danger of prolapse of the cord (see page 113).

The colour of the liquor must be observed and careful records of the fetal heart rate must be kept, to detect signs of fetal distress.

Artificial rupture of the membranes may be performed to accelerate labour; that is, when contractions have already commenced but the membranes have not ruptured spontaneously, the progress of labour is speeded up by surgical intervention.

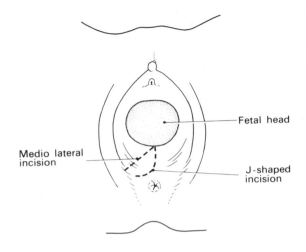

Fig. 8.3 Episiotomy.

Fetal blood sampling

Using the same techniques as for amnioscopy, a small prick is made in the fetal scalp and a drop of blood collected into a heparinized capillary tube. The blood sample is used to estimate the acidity, bicarbonate content and gas tension to detect signs of fetal distress.

Episiotomy

An episiotomy is an incision using the blunt-ended scissors through the perineum and perineal body, equivalent to a second degree tear. The perineum is infiltrated with lignocaine 0.5% to 1% if time allows. The incision may be in a lateral or medial (J-shaped) direction (Fig. 8.3). This measure accompanies forceps and breech delivery, and is employed on occasions when delivery needs to be speeded up.

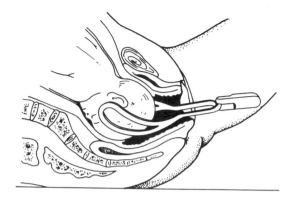

Fig. 8.4 Forceps delivery.

Forceps delivery

Obstetric forceps are designed to grasp the fetal head gently without causing injury. They can only be applied to the fetal head, and only used if the cervix is fully dilated. Traction on the forceps delivers the head (Fig. 8.4), and the body is born in the normal way. Following delivery, the baby should be observed for signs of cerebral irritation (see Chapter 13).

Vacuum (ventouse) extraction

A cup is fitted on to the presenting part, inside which a vacuum is created by suction, so that the scalp or breech is sucked up into an artificial caput known as a 'chignon'. Traction is then exerted which speeds dilatation and assists delivery (Fig. 8.5).

The chignon subsides quickly but the bruising may remain for some days. The baby is observed for signs of cerebral irritation (see Chapter 13).

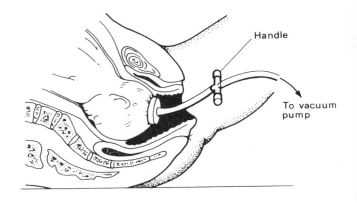

Fig. 8.5 Vacuum extraction.

Caesarean section

Caesarean section may be an emergency measure, when complications arise during labour, or it may be a planned operation, for example for patients with severe placenta praevia. An elective caesarean section carries much less risk to the fetus, who avoids the traumas of labour and vaginal delivery.

The fetus is delivered through the abdominal wall, usually via an incision into the lower segment of the uterus. The operation is performed either with a general or an epidural anaesthetic (page 100).

Preoperative preparation is detailed in Chapter 18. Post-operative care (see Chapter 19) is similar to that after any major abdominal operation, including pain relief (see page 229). Special attention is given to certain points.

Ambulation should be encouraged as early as possible because of the increased risk of thrombosis, although the patient easily becomes overtired because she has to attend to the demands of a new baby as well as to recover from her operation. Help is needed with breast-feeding because of the tender abdominal wound: the mother should be given the baby to feed him lying down when she herself is unable to get out of bed. This prevents delay in the onset of lactation.

The patient is usually discharged from hospital on about the tenth day after the operation. She is often concerned after caesarean section as to whether she can have a normal delivery in future. This is decided by the doctor who will be responsible for her care in the next pregnancy, and depends entirely on the indications for caesarean section this time. If the reasons for operation are *un*likely to recur (such as placenta praevia), then vaginal delivery is more probable than if recurrence of the problem is anticipated (such as cephalopelvic disproportion).

Manual removal of the placenta

If the whole or part of the placenta is retained in the uterus, it must be removed or haemorrhage may follow. This procedure is undertaken if there is postpartum bleeding, or if in the absence of bleeding the placenta shows no signs of separation after two hours.

A general anaesthetic is given, unless the patient already has an epidural anaesthetic, and the placenta is removed by passing a hand into the uterus and separating it from the uterine wall.

9 Physiology and Management of the Puerperium

The puerperium

The puerperium is a physiological period of six to eight weeks following childbirth when the reproductive organs return to something approaching their former size. They are always a little larger than they were before pregnancy occurred. During the early part of the puerperium the woman needs care from a midwife and this lying-in period, according to the rules of the Central Midwives Board, should be at least 10 days and up to 28 days. This care may be shared between the hospital and community midwife, or undertaken by the community midwife alone after a home confinement.

PHYSIOLOGICAL CHANGES

At the end of labour the uterus is still bulky and can be felt at the level of the umbilicus. In the next six to eight weeks this and the other structures concerned with reproduction will diminish in size. This process is called involution and is brought about by autolysis, the digestion of the extra tissues by proteolytic enzymes. Waste products are removed in the bloodstream and are excreted by the kidney.

The uterine decidua is shed rather as the endometrium in the menstrual cycle, and the discharge containing blood, shreds of membrane and decidua is called *lochia*. The lochia are red during the first two to three days, becoming reddish brown and finally pale pink in colour and serous in nature. Lochia persist for some four to eight weeks. Initially the discharge is heavier than a normal period, but the amount rapidly diminishes. Sudden red loss is abnormal and should be reported to the doctor.

It is essential that these processes take place because ligaments and muscles which fail to involute are lax and predispose to prolapse later in life (see Chapter 26).

The other main physiological change is the establishment of lactation (see Chapter 10).

MANAGEMENT

The nature of nursing changes in a postnatal ward, because patients are not normally ill and their interest is in the baby. The mother, not the nurse, is responsible for the baby's care and she instinctively guards this right closely. A nurse who tries to help by taking over the care of the baby is likely to be rejected because, however kind her motives are, she is putting the mother into a subordinate role, at the very time she needs to show her independence and confidence with the baby.

The mother wants to be seen to be a good mother now, and the nurse should therefore help her to grow in confidence. She can begin to help her by being aware of this dynamic throughout all aspects of postnatal care.

There are five aspects of care to consider when assessing the patient's needs: immediate care, physical well-being, emotional support, mother–baby relationship, and parentcraft education.

Immediate care

Bonding After delivery, parents usually experience a climax of emotions surrounding the baby: their pleasure is euphoric or, conversely, disappointment can be so acute as to cause rejection of the infant.

The first half hour after delivery is a very important time for reinforcing the bond between parents and the baby, and they should be allowed to use this time when the baby is particularly alert, to look at and cuddle and feed the baby.

Comfort The mother's main physiological need is for rest, and she should be made as comfortable as possible to enable her to relax and sleep. She should therefore be given a bedpan, bedbath, fresh nightwear and a welcome cup of tea.

Observations The temperature, pulse and blood pressure are recorded. The fundus of the uterus is examined and it should be firmly contracted at about the level of the umbilicus; the bladder should not be distended. A sterile vulval pad is given.

The care of the baby is described in Chapter 11. Once these observations are satisfactory, the patient in hospital can be transferred to the postnatal ward with the baby, or at home the patient can be left to sleep.

Physical well-being

Because the patient is not ill, she is able to attend to her physical needs herself, as long as she understands the priorities of care.

The nurse therefore has an important role in teaching patients self-care. A well-kept written record of advice given to mothers helps to prevent any one patient being given conflicting advice, as long as all staff refer to it.

Hygiene The patient is normally able to get out of bed on the day after the delivery to wash and take a shower or bath. The large placental site is an ideal breeding ground for micro-organisms, therefore good hygiene is essential to prevent

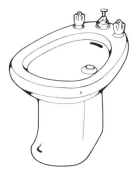

Fig. 9.1 A bidet.

infection. The perineal area should be cleansed at intervals and after every bowel action. Methods vary from hospital to hospital and include perineal swabbing, washing with soap and water and the use of the bidet (Fig. 9.1). It is the nurse's responsibility to show patients how to use the bidet, and also to ensure that baths, toilets and bidets are clean enough to be safe.

After cleansing, the area should be dried carefully and a clean vulval pad applied.

Rest The puerperium is a time when mothers need extra rest, otherwise they become extremely tired which makes even minor emotional upsets seem much worse. An afternoon rest should be encouraged, preferably lying prone as this aids drainage from the uterus and vagina. In hospital the nurse should use all her skills to promote sleep, and especially she should ensure that night-time sleep is not cut short by nursing tasks (such as waking a patient in the morning) or by other babies. At home the patient should be discouraged from undertaking household chores, and should concentrate on her own and the baby's well-being.

Exercises Postnatal exercises, often supervised by the physiotherapist, will help to restore tone to the abdominal and pelvic muscles as well as to benefit the patient as a whole (see Chapter 19).

It is essential that the nurse is aware of how much exercise the patient is taking: walking to the toilet and back with a chat at every bed can mean standing anything from a few minutes to half an hour, and in the early puerperium may lead to overtiredness.

Diet A good well-balanced diet should be taken, especially by breast-feeding mothers who often feel hungry for snacks in between mealtimes. Their diet should be increased by 500 to 1000 calories daily, and their fluid intake should be at least 2.5 litres.

Supplements of iron and extra vitamins may be given at this time. The haemoglobin level may be estimated on the third day, in order to test for anaemia.

Daily examination The patient must be examined daily by a midwife and observations recorded. This examination should be seen as an opportunity to give explanations, encouragement or reassurance to the patient, who should be enabled to use the time to discuss any problems or questions.

The temperature, pulse and blood pressure are recorded. The breasts and brassière are inspected, regardless of whether or not the mother is breast-feeding, to check that breasts are well supported and that there is no soreness or redness (see Chapter 10). The height of the uterine fundus is estimated; this should reach the symphysis pubis by the tenth postnatal day. The vaginal loss should be inspected, and the colour and amount recorded. Any perineal sutures are inspected to ensure that healing is taking place. Haematoma or infection should be reported. Sutures are usually removed on about the fifth day.

The perineum is always bruised and tender after delivery, but there should not be any haematoma or infection. Paracetamol or some mild analgesic is normally effective, and a cold compress or a saline pack will reduce any oedema. The nurse should help the patient to find a comfortable position. An air-ring cushion sometimes gives relief.

The patient should be asked if she has problems with passing urine or with bowel movements. A patient is often afraid to pass urine because of soreness of the area; also the bladder capacity is increased and sensation is decreased, so that overdistention and incomplete emptying are common. Encouragement and reassurance will help. She should have passed urine immediately before this examination and the bladder should not be palpable. There is normally a diuresis during the first two or three days as the body rids itself of excess fluid retained during pregnancy.

After the straining in the second stage of labour, constipation and haemorrhoids are common. A mild aperient may be given if necessary, which may need to be followed by a suppository on the third day. The pain of the haemorrhoids may be eased by an anaesthetic cream or suppository, and an ice pack may help to reduce their size if they are prolapsed.

Finally, the patient's legs are examined for any signs of thrombosis or phlebitis (see page 130).

Long-term care A midwife is responsible for the care of each patient for a minimum of 10 days, but if necessary for up to 28 days after delivery. She herself decides when she no longer needs to visit, once she is satisfied with all the five aspects of care.

The Health Visitor normally visits each new mother when the baby is ten days old, to introduce herself and to explain her role. She monitors the growth and development of all children under five, and is particularly concerned with preventive medicine and immunization programmes. She runs Child Health Clinics where she will give regular assessments of the baby and discuss with parents any subjects such as difficulties with feeding.

Each patient should always know how to contact her midwife and Health Visitor if she has any problems at all. She should be encouraged to attend a postnatal examination six weeks after delivery to check that the pelvic organs have returned to normal.

Emotional support

The patient may fluctuate between immense pride in her achievement at giving birth to a fear that she cannot live up to the expectations and responsibilities which motherhood involves. The nurse can help her, by recognizing the achievement (for example, by congratulating her when she meets her, and not merely taking her temperature) and by giving encouragement whenever she learns new infant skills.

Hormonal changes are often accompanied by alteration of mood, not least after delivery when a patient can find herself unusually tearful. This should pass quickly provided that care is taken to see that there are no physical causes, that she has adequate rest in a relaxed environment and that she is helped with all her difficulties.

Mother–baby relationship

Building up a relationship with her baby is a mother's priority during the puerperium, and the nurse should make as much opportunity as possible for her to do so.

The relationship develops by contact, using all the senses of sight, sound, smell, taste and touch. The baby should only be removed from the mother when absolutely necessary, thereby giving the mother the opportunity to watch her baby from her bed and learn about his behaviour. Eye-to-eye contact is very important.

The relationship deepens when a mother is increasingly involved in caring for the baby, which in turn helps her to be more confident. Separation, as when the baby needs to be in a neonatal unit, interferes with the normal relationship and the mother should be allowed to take an active part in his everyday care.

Parentcraft education

However strong the maternal instinct may be, many mothers today need to be taught skills of parentcraft because in small nuclear families girls often grow up without learning the practicalities of childcare. Unfortunately, inexperience often seems humiliating because people use standards of parentcraft skills as criteria to judge a 'good' or a 'poor' mother.

The nurse should try to understand a mother's need to be seen as a good mother. She should not only reassure her when she has learned infant skills well, but also be prepared to teach new skills without causing her to feel humiliated if she did not know already.

Subjects normally include bottle-feeding, sterilizing techniques, changing and bathing (see Chapter 11), breast-feeding (Chapter 10), and advice on contraception (Chapter 16).

COMPLICATIONS OCCURRING DURING THE PUERPERIUM

During the puerperium most women can be said to suffer some discomfort. Sometimes a patient perceives an apparently minor complication as a catastrophe. One of the most important ways the nurse can help is by listening, in order to give quiet reassurance or to notice clues when irritating symptoms are actually signs of serious complication or disorder.

Urinary complications

The bladder and urethra lie in such proximity to the birth canal that micturition is often disturbed after delivery, as after any gynaecological operations. Complications are more likely to occur after catheterization, or after a difficult operative delivery, or as a recurrence of antenatal infection (see Chapter 6). The types of complication and nursing care are described in detail in Chapter 19.

Deep vein thrombosis

There is a higher risk of deep vein thrombosis during the puerperium because of the relative haemoconcentration after pregnancy. Phlebothrombosis is more serious than thrombophlebitis because of the risk of pulmonary embolism. For this reason the patient's legs are examined daily (see 'Daily examination') and if deep vein thrombosis is diagnosed, the patient is confined to bed with the leg elevated and anticoagulant therapy is commenced. Many obstetricians prefer not to give oestrogens to suppress lactation because this further increases the risk of coagulation and thrombosis.

Uterine infection

Puerperal sepsis can follow childbirth or abortion, and is described in detail with 'Septic abortion' (Chapter 5) and 'Salpingitis' (Chapter 27).

A midwife must summon medical aid for any patient whose temperature is 38°C or over, or who has had a low-grade fever for three days. Until 1968, the infection was notifiable because puerperal sepsis used to be a major cause of maternal death, but the incidence has now declined since midwifery care has better, controlled standards and since the discovery of antibiotics.

Retained products of conception

Small shreds of membrane and sometimes a piece of placenta may be retained in the uterine cavity, which can be a serious complication because there is a risk of infection and haemorrhage. For this reason, inspection of the placenta is very important after delivery. If, when it is examined, it is thought to be incomplete, a digital exploration of the uterine cavity may be carried out under anaesthetic before the patient leaves the labour room. Incomplete membranes are usually noted but allowed to be expelled spontaneously by the uterus, usually within a day or two of delivery. Ergometrine maleate tablets (0.5 mg, three times a day for three days) are sometimes given to hasten this, but the patient should be warned that the resultant strong uterine contractions can be quite painful.

Secondary postpartum haemorrhage

Bleeding occurring from the genital tract more than 24 hours after delivery and before the end of the puerperium is known as secondary postpartum haemorrhage. It is usually caused by the retention of a piece of placenta, or in later weeks may be associated with infection.

Ergometrine maleate 0.5 mg may be given intravenously to control the bleeding initially. This is usually followed by blood transfusion and exploration of the uterine cavity.

Puerperal psychosis or neurosis

Most women are emotionally labile after delivery and one of their most pressing needs is for emotional support (see page 128). When a patient feels overwhelmed, every effort should be made to promote happy bonding with her baby, whether or not she is developing psychiatric illness. She should not be separated from the baby unless there is a clear risk of injury, and feeding or cuddling times should not be restricted. She should be given ample opportunity to rest, since tiredness worsens any feeling of depression. Happily, many emotional crises are overcome with this help, but sometimes severe psychiatric disturbance develops.

Sometimes there is a previous history of mental illness but many occur for the first time. Pregnancy does not cause mental illness but it may be the precipitating factor. The patient most likely to be affected is one whose high ideals and expectations for the baby are not realized, or who is emotionally immature or overdependent on her mother or husband. The most usual feature is insomnia, therefore any woman who is wakeful at night in the early puerperium should be observed very carefully. The patient may be unusually talkative, may be a little disjointed in speech or deluded, and in some cases there may be violent outbursts or depression and withdrawal. There is risk of injury to herself and to her baby.

The treatment depends on the severity of the condition but it is advisable for a psychiatrist to see the patient. Tranquillizers and hypnotics may be sufficient but in severe cases admission to a psychiatric hospital is necessary. Treatment may extend over several months but the prognosis is usually good.

The two greatest dangers are that the patient may be suicidal, or she may try to harm the baby, which calls for close but discreet observation and the ward should not be left unattended. The patient's husband and other members of the family need a great deal of help, support and, most of all, explanations at this time.

FURTHER READING

PRINCE, J. & ADAMS, M. (1978) *Minds, Mothers and Midwives*, Chapters 9 and 10. Edinburgh, London and New York: Churchill Livingstone.

10 Breast-feeding

Breast-feeding is natural but often involves hard work, patience, and perseverance (see Fig. 10.1). Of all the mothers who start breast-feeding, 75% of them stop within six weeks; however, recent research has shown that far fewer patients give up when they are given more support, by a midwife following up advice and showing an interest in the progress and problems. The Central Midwives Board rules that a midwife must endeavour to promote breast-feeding unless there is medical advice to the contrary.

Feeding a baby, either by breast or bottle, gives an opportunity for mother and baby to watch each other so that they can get to know one another. Breast-feeding is often a very special opportunity for this because the close contact sets the scene for intimate conversations and exploratory behaviour by both the mother and the baby. Breast-feeding has other advantages, for example the colostrum is rich in antibodies and the baby is thought to acquire passive immunity to some infections. The stools of the breast-fed baby are more acid, therefore the lactobacillus is more active in inhibiting pathogenic *Esch. coli*. Sudden infant death occurs more commonly, though not exclusively, in bottle-fed babies, but the reason for this is not yet known.

Before considering the management, it is important to understand the anatomy and physiology of the breasts, and how they are prepared for breast-feeding.

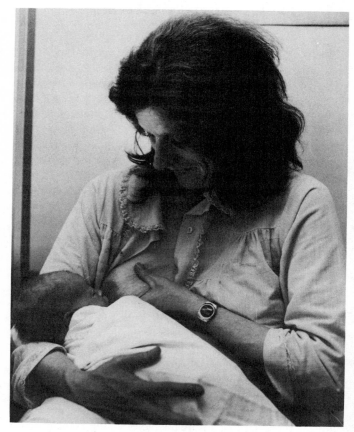

Fig. 10.1 Lactation is the natural sequel to pregnancy, but the nurse's encouragement will help when breast-feeding demands patience and determination.

Structure of the breasts

This chapter does not describe the anatomy of the whole breast (see 'Further reading'), but only those aspects directly

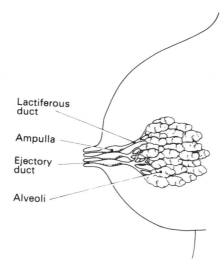

Fig. 10.2 Milk-secreting units of the breast.

related to breast-feeding which the student nurse must understand.

The breasts are composed of glandular tissue, fibrous tissue and adipose tissue. They develop at the time of the menarche (see Chapter 2) but undergo further changes during pregnancy when they are said to become mature (see 'Preparation for breastfeeding', page 136).

Each breast consists of 15–20 *lobes* which contain the milk-secreting *alveoli*. The alveoli are composed of *acini cells* which secrete the milk, and are surrounded by *myo-epithelial cells*, which are contractile and expel the milk into the ducts. The ducts widen into a small reservoir, or *ampulla*, before opening on to the surface via one of the 15–20 *ejectory ducts* (Fig. 10.2). Externally, there is a raised area of erectile tissue, the *nipple*, which is surrounded by a dark *areola*.

The breasts have a poor nerve supply and their function is

controlled by hormones. However, there is a rich blood supply, and lymphatic drainage is also extensive.

PREPARATION FOR BREAST-FEEDING

Breast changes are one of the earliest signs of pregnancy. The patient notices tenderness and tingling, which is caused by higher levels of oestrogens and progesterone enlarging and developing the milk-producing ducts and alveoli. Extra adipose tissue is laid down, and the breasts usually enlarge by at least 10 cm (4 inches) and by 1 kg in weight. This must be taken into account when buying a brassière, to give the extra support, whether or not a woman intends to breast-feed.

The breasts become more vascular with prominent veins. Pigmentation increases, first the primary areola darkens and later the skin around the primary areola becomes pigmented and is known as the secondary areola. Approximately 18 small swellings appear in the areola—enlarged sebaceous glands called *Montgomery's tubercles*, which lubricate and protect the nipple during lactation.

Colostrum is formed in the alveoli and is a fluid rich in protein and antibodies. If the patient squeezes the nipple gently, she can see a drop of this opalescent white fluid; this usually encourages her to see how natural breast-feeding is, and also helps her to become used to handling the breasts and nipple.

PHYSIOLOGY OF MILK PRODUCTION

It is important for the nurse to understand the various mechanisms which work together to produce milk, in order to give appropriate advice and simply to be able to explain to mothers what is happening to them.

Milk production

Prolactin During pregnancy the high levels of oestrogens and progesterone act as a brake which prevents large quantities of milk from being produced. As soon as the placenta is delivered, this brake is taken away, and as the levels of circulating oestrogens and progesterone fall, the milk-producing hormone *prolactin* is produced. If the patient does not wish to breast-feed, the breasts may become uncomfortably full for a couple of days (see 'Suppression of lactation'). If, however, the patient does wish to breast-feed, she can augment this initial supply by giving the greatest stimulus to milk production—suckling.

Demand–supply The initial supply of milk will dry up unless other stimulation is given to tell the body to continue production. The only other stimulation is by the baby suckling. Suckling stimulates the nerves leading to the pituitary gland which produces more prolactin.

This allows a delicate balance, such that a mother always produces a supply to match her baby's need; so, for example, the supply changes according to the demands of a newborn baby, a four-month-old baby, or even twins, all of whom can be entirely breast-fed.

Unfortunately, artificial interference (such as giving a bottle) disturbs this balance, and can cause mothers to produce less milk (Fig. 10.3). Many mothers mistakenly reduce their own milk supply by giving the baby a bottle instead of a breast-feed: this causes less prolactin to be released, which causes a subsequent reduction in milk supply. Therefore, a patient who is afraid that she has insufficient milk should *never* be advised to give a bottle, unless she wants to suppress lactation, but she should allow the baby to suckle more at the breast.

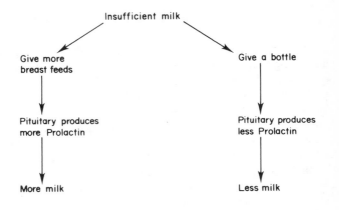

Fig. 10.3 Diagram to show that the supply of milk meets the demand by the baby suckling.

Release of milk

Let-down reflex (Fig. 10.4) When the baby suckles, a nerve impulse is sent to the posterior pituitary. In response, the pituitary releases the hormone oxytocin, which causes contraction of the myoepithelial cells and milk spurts out. This is called the let-down reflex, and is felt by the woman as a tingling in the breast. The maximum milk flow can take up to three minutes, therefore if suckling time is restricted, the baby will be removed from the breast before he has benefited from this supply.

The let-down reflex can be inhibited by circumstances, for example fatigue, or anxiety, or if a patient is made to feel nervous by the apparently judgemental eyes of an onlooker. She can be helped at this stage by being made really comfortable, free from time pressure, and with the reassurance that she *is* doing the right thing.

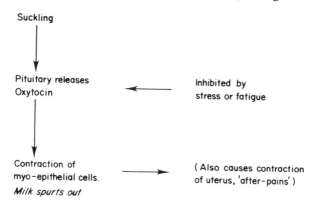

Fig. 10.4 Diagram to show the let-down reflex.

Oxytocin released during the let-down reflex also travels in the bloodstream to the uterus, causing contraction, and many women complain of 'after pains' whilst breast-feeding.

Foremilk Before the let-down reflex occurs, the baby receives the fluid stored in the ampullae (see Fig. 10.2), called *foremilk*. This is very thirst quenching and low in calories: the milk becomes richer as the feed progresses.

The baby obtains the milk by the driving action of his gums around the base of the areola, which compresses the ampullae and forces milk out. If the baby takes only the nipple into his mouth, he will get no milk and moreover it predisposes to very sore nipples.

MANAGEMENT OF BREAST-FEEDING

An understanding of the physiology is extremely important because adequate milk production is dependent upon the appropriate application of this knowledge to breast-feeding patients. A nurse should never give any advice until she understands the related physiology. The primipara needs very practical advice and support and the nurse should be at hand in case she is needed.

Before feeding, both mother and baby should be made comfortable, so that each one can concentrate. The mother should empty her bladder, wash her hands and then find somewhere that she feels relaxed to feed—a low chair, or a sofa, or bed (Fig. 10.5). The baby, too, may have his napkin changed but he will be unable to settle if he is really screaming with hunger. It is always beneficial if the mother is given time to love and admire the baby for a few minutes because this has a calming effect on them both.

The baby's rooting reflex causes him to turn naturally towards any stimulus to the cheek, therefore when the mother is ready, she should stroke his cheek gently with the exposed nipple and he will root towards it. Correct positioning on the nipple is essential to prevent sore nipples: the whole areola should be well into the mouth, above the tongue, so that the gums can perform the essential driving action. The baby should be supported securely such that he does not pull on the breast. This is especially true at the end of a feed when he should be removed from the nipple either by pressing on his chin, or by inserting a finger between his lips and the breast, so releasing the vacuum.

At the end of the feed, the baby should be sat upright to bring up wind, although breast-fed babies have less wind than bottle-fed ones. The mother should dry the nipples and apply a lanolin cream or protective spray. The straps of her brassière should be adjusted frequently to match the changing size and weight of the breasts.

At subsequent feeds, the baby starts on alternate sides, because the first breast taken is the one more thoroughly emptied. The baby should normally be allowed to suckle

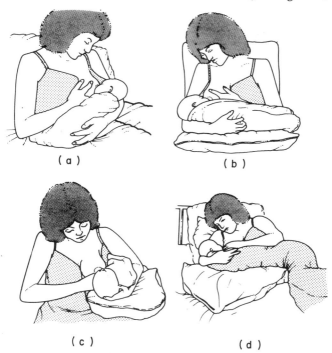

Fig. 10.5 Positions for breast-feeding. (a) Sitting up in bed, back well
supported; (b) Sitting on a chair, back supported; (c) Suitable
position following a Caesarean; (d) Feeding lying down.

until he is satisfied, as long as he is drinking well from the
breast.

The colostrum produced in the first few days is rich in
nutrients as well as protective antibodies, and there is no
need to give additional feeds from a bottle. Most babies have
a store of energy at birth, which runs out by about the fourth
day when they want to feed very often. This coincides with

the time when the mother's breasts are very full, so the baby's extra feeding relieves the mother's uncomfortably full breasts.

Breast-feeding is hard work physically, and the mother must replace the calories she is spending by eating nourishing foods and by taking ample fluids. Most women naturally feel more hungry and thirsty, and often take some of the extra fluids at the time of the baby's feed. Any ward routine in hospital must consider their need for additional snacks during the day or night.

PROBLEMS ASSOCIATED WITH BREAST-FEEDING

Insufficient milk Many women fear that they have insufficient milk, partly because they cannot see how much the baby is taking. If the baby seems unsatisfied, the feed should be supervised to make sure that he is fixed correctly and obtaining milk, not just chewing at the nipple. If he is suckling well, then the problem will soon right itself (see 'Physiology: Demand–supply'), as long as the mother's diet is adequate and the neurohormone reflex is not inhibited by overtiredness or anxiety (see 'Physiology: Let-down reflex').

Sore nipples Breast-feeding should not be painful, apart from the initial discomfort when the baby first fixes on to the breast. Sore and cracked nipples should normally be prevented by never allowing the baby to drag on the breast (see 'Management of breast-feeding'). If the baby is not being fed often enough, he will suck more strongly, because he will be so hungry.

If soreness does develop, the next feed should be supervised to ensure that the baby is being supported without pulling on the breast, and to check that the mother is caring for her nipples adequately. A cracked nipple must be rested and milk expressed by hand, and a spray or ointment may be given to aid healing.

Engorged breasts The breasts can become engorged with fluid on about the second day when the blood flow increases, and they become bluish in colour, oedematous, tense and very uncomfortable. This is not relieved by feeding but they often feel more comfortable being bathed with very hot and very cold water.

Milk engorgement occurs on around the fourth day, when the milk supply increases dramatically. This type of engorgement is partly relieved by feeding the baby, although if the nipple becomes flattened the baby finds great difficulty in suckling. The patient gains great relief if milk is expressed thoroughly, once, until the breast is empty.

Both venous and milk engorgement can occur whether or not the patient is breast-feeding. After expression the discomfort is helped by giving extra support such as with a breast binder, although analgesics such as paracetamol may also be indicated.

Failure to breast-feed Sometimes numerous problems all build up, which are as individual as each baby, and mothers often become confused between all the advice from the midwife, friends and family. Most problems can be overcome, but if a mother does decide to stop breast-feeding, she may feel that *she* has failed.

Feeling a failure gives a bad start to motherhood, and the nurse should try to reassure her that the baby most needs her, to enjoy the love and security she brings. Breast-feeding should be a help, rather than a handicap, for this kind of relationship.

Mastitis Mastitis is infection of the breast, which is usually localized because fibrous tissue called septae divide each breast into 15 or 20 lobes. The breast is painful and on examination it has a flushed area, is hard and hot to the touch. The axillary glands may be swollen and the temperature and pulse raised.

A specimen of milk is sent for culture and the appropriate antibiotic prescribed. Feeding is discontinued from the affected breast which should be emptied by hand and the milk discarded. Once the infection has subsided feeding may be resumed.

If mastitis is not treated early, an abscess may develop.

Breast abscess An abscess must be incised and drained in theatre under a general anaesthetic. Arrangements are usually made for the baby to be kept beside his mother during her stay in hospital.

SUPPRESSION OF LACTATION

Milk is normally produced in response to stimuli (see 'Physiology'), therefore if the stimulus of suckling is not made, the supply of milk gradually diminishes. However, if a mother does not intend to breast-feed, the normal process can be speeded up. Bromocryptine inhibits prolactin, as does oestrogen, but the latter is given less frequently now because it carries an increased risk of deep vein thrombosis.

The breasts can become engorged despite treatment; see 'Problems associated with breast-feeding'.

FURTHER READING

JACKSON, S. (1979) *Anatomy and Physiology for Nurses*. London: Baillière Tindall.

11 The Normal Baby and Parentcraft Education

The baby has overcome many hazards during its passage through the birth canal but possibly the greatest of them all is its transition from fetal life to that of a healthy newborn infant. Birth involves a very rapid change from the warm, sheltered life of the uterus, to a cold uncertain world outside. It is suggested that the more gently the baby is introduced to this environment, the more easily and contentedly he will adapt to it (see 'Further reading').

The nurse's aim when she is called to give first aid to a baby immediately after delivery should be to make the environment as free as possible from complicating factors such as cold, thus protecting him so that the essential physiological changes are not impeded.

Physiological changes

After birth the baby no longer has the placenta to perform vital functions, so immediately the cord is cut the lungs must come into use and the route of the blood must change.

Inspiration is thought to be initiated by a combination of factors. As the fetal chest passes through the vagina it is squeezed and this probably forces liquor from the alveoli into the respiratory tract from where it either drains spontaneously or it is aspirated by the nurse. Secondly, the air of a room is colder than the internal environment and this acts as a stimulus; thirdly, carbon dioxide in the blood has been slightly raised during labour. These factors stimulate the respiratory centre and the baby inspires, fills the lungs with air and so alters the pressure within the thorax.

The severing of the fetal cord stops blood flow in the umbilical vessels, the hypogastric arteries and the ductus venosus (see Fig. 3.16). This reduces the pressure of blood reaching the right atrium, and the pressure on the right side of the heart falls. The lung substance stretches on inspiration and with it the blood vessels stretch, which pulls blood from the right ventricle into the pulmonary circulation, further reducing right-sided pressure. The pulmonary return to the left atrium causes pressure on the left side to rise and eventually it exceeds the pressure on the right side and the foramen ovale closes. The blood from the right ventricle finds it easier to pass to the lungs now and tends to rush past the ductus arteriosus, so this flow gradually ceases and later the structure becomes a small ligament. The ductus venosus and hypogastric arteries eventually become ligaments. The terminal capillaries are not well formed in the newborn and the extremities tend to be blue.

On rare occasions the ductus arteriosus fails to occlude and, because systemic pressure is higher than pulmonary pressure, reverse flow occurs from the aorta to the pulmonary artery causing pulmonary congestion.

The baby's temperature is unstable initially and it takes the heat-regulating centre some days to adjust. The newborn cannot shiver and relies on his surroundings to maintain his temperature. For this reason he should be wrapped warmly and should never be undressed for bathing in a cold room.

The gastrointestinal tract begins to function normally. The passage of meconium demonstrates that the lower bowel is patent, whereas the passing of a brown changing stool shows that digested milk is passing down and the whole tract is patent. For this reason, observation of the infant's stools is important.

The kidneys normally excrete urine whilst in its utero but this increases after birth. The ability to concentrate urine is poor in the first months of life, causing relatively large quantities to be passed.

Priorities of care

The initial establishment of respiration, cutting of the cord and, in hospital, labelling the baby, are the responsibility of the midwife who delivers. Further care such as cleaning and weighing the baby should not be rushed, because more important is the relationship between the baby and his parents.

A baby is especially alert during the first half hour after delivery and this corresponds with the new parents' delight and their desire to have a good look and admire. This time can be one when a very special bond is initiated and should never be stolen by staff, for example by removing the baby from the parents, except for urgent treatment or care.

First inspection of the baby

Certain observations of the baby should be carried out, either beside the parents if they want to watch, or in another warm room (21°C, 70°F) whilst the mother is resting.

The nurse should note the colour of the baby and whether the respirations are normal: if not this could denote some cardiac or respiratory abnormality. She should look for any obvious defects in the shape of the head, and feel the sutures and fontanelles gently. The anterior fontanelle is fairly large, diamond shaped and soft to the touch and should be neither depressed nor bulging. She should observe the degree of moulding and note any swellings on the head. The ears, arms, hands, fingers, feet, legs and toes are examined very carefully to note any deformities such as extra or absent digits. Paralysis, talipes or meningocele may be detected at this stage. Certain other defects are less obvious, for example cleft palate may only be seen if the mouth is examined in a good light, and excessive mucus in the mouth may indicate a blind end to the oesophagus (oesophageal atresia). The baby's rectal temperature is taken gently and recorded. If the thermometer meets resistance, the anus may be imperforate.

These observations are often carried out whilst giving the baby skin care, either by bathing him or by simple cleansing with cotton wool. All traces of blood should be removed but the greasy covering, the *vernix caseosa*, need not be removed except from skin folds such as the neck, groin and axillae. If this is difficult, a little arachis oil on a swab will be effective.

Subsequent observations

Unlike the adult, the baby cannot explain all his needs verbally and the nurse has to rely on her observations in order to know if he is comfortable. It is vital to remember that the condition of the baby can change very rapidly and constant observation is necessary if the baby's condition is not satisfactory.

General appearance The colour of the baby should be noted. Cyanosis may indicate a cardiac condition, pallor could indicate anaemia, and jaundice may be serious depending on the time of occurrence (see Chapter 13). The baby tends to lie in a curled up position as in its utero, and limb extension or rigidity is not normal.

Sleep Babies do not distinguish night from day and tend to waken at intervals when they are uncomfortable, because they are hungry, have wind or sometimes they simply seem to want cuddling. They normally sleep for about 20 of the 24 hours, although it is now thought that sleep patterns are inborn and that wakeful nights are not the fault of training by parents.

Stools The type of stool changes in the first week after birth.

Meconium During the intrauterine period the gut is full of meconium, which is a sticky, dark greenish stool composed of gastric and intestinal juices, liquor amnii, cells and debris from the gut lining. It is passed for about three days after birth.

Changing stool The meconium becomes light brown in colour. This change is evidence that the whole gastrointestinal tract is patent because digested milk is added to meconium.

Normal stool Finally, by about the fifth day, the stool takes on a curdy bright yellow appearance. The number of stools in 24 hours is variable, usually four to five.

Any deviations from this should be reported. Malaena may occur in the newborn and is usually detected by its odour. Green stools indicate some dietary defect.

Micturition It is important to note when the infant passes urine, particularly with a boy. It is not uncommon for the baby to pass urine at birth when he comes into contact with the cold environment, and if a record is not kept of this, anxiety may be caused. Failure to pass urine may indicate urethral obstruction or renal agenesis.

Skin The skin of the neonate is usually very soft, having been protected by the vernix against the effect of being immersed constantly in liquor. After birth, however, the vernix is removed and unless a protective cream such as zinc and castor oil is used, the napkin area suffers from frequent contact with moisture. Alternatively, one-way liners help to keep the skin of the buttocks dry.

Any rashes or pustules should be noted and reported because of the danger of infection. The eyes may be cleansed daily or left alone, unless there is some discharge. Variation of care is dependent upon the individual unit concerned.

The umbilicus requires a daily toilet with sterile swabs and spirit to clean and dry the cord and surrounding area. Hexachlorophene powder is then applied as an antiseptic and drying agent. The cord should separate spontaneously about the fifth day. Any moistness or odour should be reported.

Weight The baby's body reserves are utilized and meconium and urine are passed which both contribute to the weight loss during the first three to four days. After this, there is a steady weight gain and most babies regain their birth weight within two weeks.

The birth weight is usually doubled by the sixth month, and trebled at one year. The mother should be reassured that the weight of the baby is only one of several signs of a healthy baby, but that physical well-being and contentment are equally important.

Neonatal abilities

The neonate has many abilities about which the nurse can educate parents so that they can understand his behaviour better and provide a wide range of experiences to stimulate him. If a baby is in an incubator, it is especially important to communicate with him by looking, talking and listening to him (Fig. 12.1).

Reflexes The baby can react with certain reflexes such as the rooting, sucking, swallowing (see Chapter 10), grasp, primitive walking, and moro reflex. Each of these is explained in a paediatric textbook.

A normal baby also communicates by crying, which is often a sign of need such as for food or security.

Perception The baby can perceive his environment and selects some aspects as more interesting than others. He can, for example, ignore some noises and stop crying for others. He perceives by looking, hearing, smelling and touching.

Looking Visual exploration is an important way of learning and getting to know the world. A neonate can focus on the human face and can even recognize his mother's face by one week. He should therefore be held where he is enabled to look around him.

Hearing A baby can appreciate rhythm, pitch and loudness and can become accustomed to irrelevant noises.

Smelling A neonate can distinguish his own mother's milk from another milk, by his sense of smell.

Touching The baby experiences the world through touch, and parents should therefore not be prevented from handling, stroking, rocking and cuddling.

PARENTCRAFT EDUCATION

New parents are very ready to learn the practicalities of caring for their baby. However, sometimes they appear to be unreceptive to teaching, because they are afraid that to ask for help will make them seem like poor parents. To avoid this, the nurse should show each mother the recognition of her unique position as mother, without talking down to her.

Parentcraft means giving advice to help parents to make

their own decision. Care should be taken to avoid giving instructions which conflict with another's advice, for example with that given in antenatal classes. Often a mother is encouraged by being commended on what she knows, rather than constantly being shown her failures.

Parentcraft teaching may be given to individuals or groups. The nurse should remember that a mother's concentration is poor at this time, therefore advice must always be clear. Too much information is as confusing as too little.

The subjects taught vary, but usually include bottle-feeding, sterilization techniques, breast-feeding, and a demonstration of bathing a baby.

Bottle-feeding Mothers should be shown how to prepare and give the baby artificial milk. They should be helped to understand the dangerous pitfalls, such as of inaccurate measurements or of inadequate sterilization, and be taught how to avoid them.

All packets or tins of modified milk give instructions on how to mix the formula, and these instructions *must* be followed exactly. It cannot be emphasized too strongly that when measuring the dried milk, the correct amount of dried powder must be measured by using the correct scoop, supplied with each packet. If too much formula is used in proportion to water, the baby will be thirsty and could even suffer from *hypernatraemia*.

Several bottles of milk may be prepared at one time, and then stored in a refrigerator ready for use during the day or night. The amount of milk a baby will drink is calculated according to his weight, although at some times he will take more than at other times because appetite varies during the day. Normally a baby takes 3 oz (85 ml) of milk per pound (0.45 kg) of body weight per 24 hours. A 7-lb (3.2 kg) baby will thus take about 21 oz, (595 ml) in 24 hours.

Bottle-feeding can be almost as intimate as breast-feeding.

The baby should be given a bottle by someone who has the time to enjoy the physical closeness and eye contact.

Cow's milk is unsuitable for babies unless it is modified. Many milk foods are modified to make their composition as near to human milk as possible, as shown in Table 11.1.

Sterilization of utensils All the baby's feeding utensils must be sterilized for two reasons. First, babies have little or no immunity against bacteria, and second, warm milk is an ideal breeding ground for bacteria which will then be ingested and can rapidly cause fatal gastroenteritis.

The utensils to be sterilized include bottles, caps, teats, measuring jug and spoon. They can either be boiled for 15 minutes, or submerged in a solution of hypochlorite for 2 hours. Instructions for making the solution are given on the sterilant, and parents should be given a demonstration and told to change the solution daily.

Breast-feeding See Chapter 10.

Table 11.1. Composition of human, cow's and modified cow's milk

Component	Human breast milk	Cow's milk	Modified cow's milk (SMA)
Carbohydrate*	6.8	4.9	7.2
Fat*	4.5	3.7	3.6
Protein*	1.1	3.5	1.5
Sodium (mmol/litre)	7.0	22.0	7.0
Phosphorus (mg/litre)	140.0	920.0	330.0
Calcium (mg/litre)	340.0	1170.0	445.0

* per 100 ml of formula.

Bathing a baby Bathing a baby is described in full because the procedure differs little between the various Health Districts.

Before bathing, the nursery should be prepared, all windows closed to prevent draughts and the room temperature not less than 21°C (70°F). Towels, swabs, vest, gown, napkin and pin should be placed ready for use, preferably over a warm radiator. The baby is then undressed except for his napkin which should not be removed until after the face has been cleansed in order to minimize infection (and mess!).

The baby is wrapped in a warm, soft towel and the face and hair are attended to first. Bathing is not a sterile procedure but in order to avoid introducing infection, each swab is used once only, using water from a clean container and not the bath. In hospital the swabs have usually been sterilized, but at home the mother may use clean cotton wool or a face flannel kept for this purpose.

The eyes are swabbed with clean warm water, swabbing from the nose outwards. The face is then washed and dried with a swab. The hair is washed using shampoo and then rinsed with clear water, by supporting the head with the left hand and tucking the body under the arm.

If a solution of babybath is to be used, this should not be added until after the hair has been rinsed. The head is dried with a towel using the flat of the hand. The towel is unwrapped and the baby's body is lathered all over with soap. The baby is then immersed in the bath, his head being supported by the nurse's left arm and his arm being held by her left hand whilst she uses her right hand to rinse off the soap. The baby should be allowed to enjoy a good kick in the bath.

The baby is lifted out and placed face downward on the towel to dry his back. The baby is then turned over and the front dried. The vest may be put on for warmth before petroleum jelly or cream is applied to protect the buttocks.

The napkin is put on; if pins are used the nurse should place her fingers between the pin and the baby whilst inserting it, and place it crosswise, not lengthwise, in case it opens and injures the baby. Lastly, the baby is dressed and given a reassuring cuddle.

FURTHER READING

KELNAR, C.J.H. & HARVEY, D. (1981) *The Sick Newborn Baby*, Chapter 4. London: Baillière Tindall.

LEBOYER, F. (1977) *Birth Without Violence*. London: Fontana/Collins.

PRINCE, J. & ADAMS, M. (1978) *Minds, Mothers and Midwives*, Chapter 4. Edinburgh, London and New York: Churchill Livingstone.

12 The Premature Baby

A premature baby usually has a low birth weight, but prematurity must be distinguished from the other cause of low birth weight, that is, light-for-dates babies.

A *low-birth-weight baby* is a baby who weighs 2500 g or less at birth, irrespective of gestational age.

A *premature baby* (preterm baby) is one born before 37 completed weeks of gestation. The degree of maturity influences the chance of survival and, although legally an infant is viable after the 28th week, in fact the dangers of prematurity decrease the later the baby is born.

A *light-for-dates baby* is one whose birth weight is below the 10th centile for its estimated gestational age. A baby is light for dates if there was intrauterine malnutrition or growth retardation, such as when the mother smoked during pregnancy.

CHARACTERISTICS OF THE PREMATURE BABY

The premature baby is easily recognized, the head is large in proportion to the body and he has a small triangular face with a pointed chin and worried expression. If very small he may be slow to open his eyes. The sutures and fontanelles are widely spaced, and the skull bones soft. The skin is red and wrinkled because there is little subcutaneous fat, and he is covered with a soft downy hair called lanugo. The limbs are thin, the nails short, the chest small and soft, the abdomen large and nipples poorly developed. The genitalia are small and the testes may not have descended into the scrotum. The baby may be feeble and drowsy and the sucking reflex may be poor. The cerebral centres are underdeveloped with the result that the circulatory system may be unstable and there is poor control of body temperature. The respiratory centre is not fully developed and the baby may have cyanotic attacks, especially after feeding. There is little or no immunity to infection and a greater tendency to bleeding than in the mature baby.

CARE OF THE PREMATURE BABY

The nursing care of the premature baby is of vital importance and his chance of survival depends on the care he receives. Care will be supervised by a paediatrician and the baby is usually admitted to a special care nursery.

In the early stages, continuous observation is necessary and a record must be kept of colour, rate and regularity of respiration, whether there is any rib recession, temperature of the baby and incubator, pulse rate, whether any twitchings or fits occur.

In addition to giving physical care, it is vital to meet the very different needs of the mother, of the baby, and of them both together as they establish their relationship.

Problems of prematurity

The problems of prematurity may be identified as follows.

1. Establishment and maintenance of adequate respiration.
2. Establishment of adequate feeding and prevention of dehydration.
3. Maintenance of body temperature without restricting excursions.
4. Prevention of infection.
5. Promoting the parent–baby bond when there is physical separation.

Respiration The lungs of the premature baby are immature and one of the greatest dangers to the baby's life is *respiratory distress syndrome*. The lungs cannot expand fully and the infant becomes hypoxaemic. The main signs, which appear within four hours of delivery, are an audible expiratory grunt, sternal recession and tachypnoea (over 60 breaths per minute).

The baby is nursed in a warm incubator where the maximum humidity is achieved. Oxygen is usually required by continuous positive airways pressure, either via a head box or an endotracheal tube. This pressure is necessary to prevent lung collapse.

Blood samples must be taken to measure gas tension, acidity and bicarbonate content. Too high an oxygen tension in the blood causes *retrolental fibroplasia* which results in blindness. Depending on the blood results, the paediatrician may order intravenous fluids such as glucose and bicarbonate. These correct the blood chemistry and relieve the asphyxia, and at the same time prevent acidosis. In the newborn, intravenous fluids are usually given through a cannula inserted into the umbilical vein.

Feeding The action of feeding from a bottle is often easier for the baby than breast-feeding, but the mother is encouraged to express her milk into a sterile container and this can be given to the baby. Occasionally human breast milk is donated to special care baby units, called milk banks, but if milk from such a unit is not available, modified cow's milk preparations may be substituted.

The premature baby requires a higher calorie intake than the mature baby (150 to 200 calories per kg of body weight per day). Some babies cannot actually manage the volume of fluid this entails, so extra protein such as Casilan may be added.

If the baby is too weak to suck at all, a Jacques' catheter

moistened with water may be introduced through the nose or mouth. Paediatricians may vary in their opinions as to whether the tube is passed at each feed or left in position for long periods. The nurse must never pass an intragastric tube without being supervised by a trained person, and if one is left in position the baby must be under constant observation. The close proximity of the oesophagus and trachea makes it very easy for fluid to spill over into the lungs and cause asphyxia or pneumonia if the tube moves out of position.

Feeding may be two- or three-hourly throughout the 24 hours, the night feeds gradually being omitted as the baby gains in weight and maturity.

Temperature The temperature of the nursery should not be less than 21°C (70°F) and may be higher. Many babies will be nursed in an incubator whose temperature is maintained at 32°C (90°F). This allows for control of temperature and humdity and gives maximum scope for observation. The baby is nursed naked in the incubator because this relieves the chest of the weight of clothes and helps respiration.

Infection Prevention of infection is easier in a special care unit, aided by the incubator. Personnel entering the unit must wear gowns and masks and wash their hands carefully before handling the baby. Disposable towels, napkins and other utensils help to avoid cross-infection. Anyone with the slightest sign of infection, such as a cold or boil, is not admitted to the nursery. The slightest sign of pyrexia, slowness to feed or deterioration in colour will be regarded as a serious sign, investigated and treated with the appropriate antibiotic.

Bonding The protection which an incubator provides also acts as a barrier against normal human contact (see Fig. 12.1). One of the nurse's duties is therefore to encourage

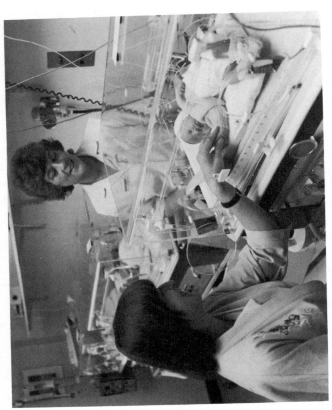

Fig. 12.1 The protection which an incubator provides also acts as a barrier against normal human contact. The nurse can encourage parents to stimulate the baby by touch and by eye-to-eye

patients to stimulate the baby by touch and by eye-to-eye contact. This problem is discussed in more detail on page 162.

Other hazards of prematurity Certain other hazards are likely to occur in the premature baby.

Physiological jaundice This is common, and the serum bilirubin may rise to dangerous levels and require treatment (Chapter 13).

Anaemia The fetus lays down its store of iron in the last four weeks of pregnancy, so it is unlikely that the premature baby has much reserve. A liquid preparation of iron is introduced about the fourth week to help overcome this.

Bleeding Because of the immaturity of the liver there are often clotting defects in the premature baby. A vitamin K preparation, phytomenadione (Konakion) 1 mg, is given by injection soon after birth.

Progress As the baby grows he will be removed from the incubator to a cot in a slightly cooler nursery and the mother will be taught how to bath and care for him, and breast-feeding may be commenced if her lactation is well established. Premature babies are usually discharged when they weigh 2.5 kg if their condition is satisfactory.

FURTHER READING

KELNAR, C.J.H. & HARVEY, D. (1981) *The Sick Newborn Baby*, Chapters 5 and 6. London: Baillière Tindall.

13 Disorders of the Newborn

Any disorder of the newborn baby, however small, changes the interaction between the baby and his parents, partly because the parents cannot enter fully into the normal sense of achievement and wonder at a perfect infant. More specifically, the interaction changes because mother and baby may be separated whilst treatment is given, and early separation can inhibit the bonding of mother and baby.

Management of the baby's condition is usually planned and carried out by the paediatrician, with nurses who specialize in the care of neonates. The student nurse can give special care to the postnatal mother by encouraging her to visit her baby, taking her in a wheelchair if necessary. She can enable the mother to talk about her worries, for example by showing interest in the baby's progress whenever she has visited the special care baby unit: listening is a very important part of caring (Fig. 13.1). The midwife may also be required to help with practicalities such as expressing breast milk for nasogastric feeds.

There are many abnormal conditions which may affect the newborn. A few of the most important disorders will be described in detail, and a short summary of others will be given. Further details may be found in a textbook of paediatrics.

Asphyxia

The transition at birth from placental oxygenation to the use of the lungs may be difficult (see 'Physiological changes',

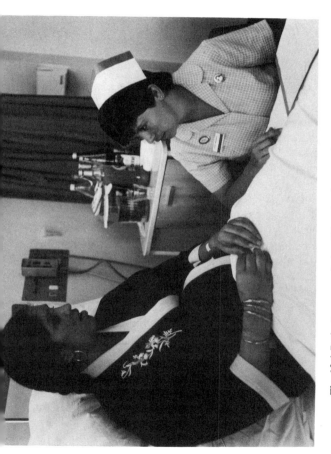

Fig. 13.1 Patients are people too. Listening is a very important part of caring.

Chapter 11). Mucus or blood may block the air passages, muscles may be weak, or there may be some hindrance to the passage of gases in the alveoli. Any of these conditions leads to asphyxia.

When the baby is born the degree of asphyxia may be mild or severe.

Mild asphyxia The face and extremities are blue but muscle tone is good and the heart beat strong. The air passages are aspirated with a mucus extractor and some form of peripheral stimulation help, such as flicking the feet and drying the baby with a towel. The baby usually responds by gasping and crying.

Severe asphyxia The colour is grey, the heart beat is irregular, weak or even absent and the baby is limp with poor muscle tone. Treatment is urgent and the nurse can give first-aid help by clearing the air passages and giving mouth-to-mouth resuscitation or preferably oxygen by a face mask or neonatal inflating bag. Only positive pressure methods of artificial respiration can be used if the lungs have not yet expanded.

Once the paediatrician arrives he can pass an endotracheal tube to give oxygen under pressure. Once respiration is

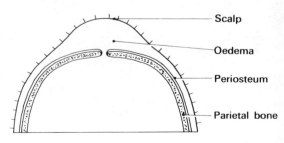

Fig. 13.2 Caput succedaneum.

established the parents should be allowed a reassuring cuddle with their baby, who should subsequently be observed closely in his cot for at least 24 hours.

Swellings of the head

There are two main causes of swellings on the baby's head at birth. Because the two conditions are so similar, yet take such different times to resolve, it is essential that the parents are not given wrong information. They will lose confidence in the nurse if they are assured that the swelling will disappear in a few hours and it is still present weeks later.

Caput succedaneum Caput succedaneum is a bluish swelling on the baby's head which is present at birth (Fig. 13.2). It always lies over the presenting part, having been caused by the pressure of the dilating cervix which impeded venous return.

The parents should be told that this type of swelling disappears within 24 hours, and that the baby's head will resume a normal shape.

Cephalhaematoma Cephalhaematoma is a swelling which may be present at birth or may occur later, it tends to increase in size and is due to bleeding under the periosteum (Fig. 13.3). The cause is trauma during birth which has separated

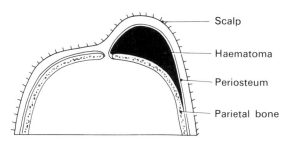

Fig. 13.3 **Cephalhaematoma.**

a small area of periosteum and precipitated bleeding. As it lies under the periosteum it is limited to a single bone and does not cross a suture, it may however be bilateral.

A haematoma will take time to be absorbed and the swelling may be present for six to eight weeks after delivery. The following comparison may be helpful.

Caput succedaneum	*Cephalhaematoma*
Oedema	Haematoma
Caused by pressure	Caused by trauma
Present at birth	Appears later
Tends to reduce in size	Tends to increase in size
Pits on pressure	Does not pit on pressure
May cross a suture	Cannot cross a suture
Disappears in 24 hours	Persists for 6 to 8 weeks

Cerebral irritation

Cerebral irritation may occur after prolonged intrauterine asphyxia, after a rapid or traumatic delivery which caused the rupture of small blood vessels. The baby is restless, and, if disturbed, reacts with a shrill cry.

The head should be raised slightly above the feet and the cot placed in a quiet area away from a direct bright light. Constant observation is necessary and if a fit occurs it may be of great value if the nurse notices where it began and the order of movement of the limbs. A sedative such as phenobarbitone by intramuscular injection may be ordered until the condition subsides.

The parents should be told that the baby should be handled specially gently for a few days, and that other visitors should not be allowed to lift him from the cot.

Jaundice

Jaundice is a symptom, not a disease, and is often seen in the newborn. There are several causes of this condition.

Physiological jaundice The so-called physiological jaundice is due to normal breakdown of red cells which occurs in all babies after birth. In some of them, and particularly in the premature baby, the rate of breakdown is greater than the rate of elimination of bile pigments from the bloodstream, and this accounts for the jaundice which appears on the third or fourth day.

Treatment It is thought that extra fluids (breast-feeds or sterile water) may help physiological jaundice. The serum bilirubin level is estimated by blood test. If the serum bilirubin rises above 250 mmol/litre, phototherapy may be used. This is a blue spectrum of light which converts fat-soluble bilirubin to water-soluble bilirubin which can be excreted. Special attention must be given to temperature control, fluid loss and skin care during phototherapy.

Haemolytic jaundice Haemolysis of red cells due to iso-immunization to the Rhesus factor or the ABO groups will result in jaundice, the most common type being Rhesus incompatibility (see below).

Obstructive jaundice Obstructive jaundice is a rare condition and is caused by congenital obliteration of the bile ducts. It is eventually fatal.

Rhesus isoimmunization

Jaundice can be one sign of Rhesus incompatibility, a haemolytic anaemia brought about by the action of maternal anti-Rhesus antibodies. It is a serious, even fatal, condition but can now be prevented very simply (see 'Prophylaxis').

As with other immunizations, the presence of foreign-protein antigen stimulates the formation of antibodies which break down the antigen. A Rhesus-positive person carries the antigen, and a Rhesus-negative person does not: if any antigens enter the circulation of a Rhesus-negative person, antibodies are formed. This is important in relation to pregnancy because isoimmunity can occur when the mother is Rhesus negative and the baby Rhesus positive. The mother produces antibodies whenever fetal red cells escape into her circulation—namely, after a placental bleed, however small, and after separation of the placenta. Rhesus isoimmunization is therefore rare in the first pregnancy because it cannot occur until *after* fetal cells have escaped into the maternal circulation.

Some maternal antibodies, once formed against fetal antigen, pass across the placenta into the fetal bloodstream and destroy the antigen and red blood cells. This leads to anaemia, which may progress to a condition called hydrops fetalis when there is severe oedema and enlargement of the liver and spleen. This eventually results in intrauterine death.

Jaundice at birth is rare, because the maternal liver usually deals with excess bilirubin from broken down red blood cells; but it appears in the first few hours after delivery. The baby's immature liver cannot convert the fat-soluble bilirubin to water-soluble, therefore unchanged bilirubin is deposited in fatty tissue including vital areas of the brain. The presence of bilirubin in brain cells is known as kernicterus and leads to convulsions and cerebral palsy.

Investigations Antenatally, at the booking clinic, the maternal blood and Rhesus group are determined and if the blood is Rhesus negative, further specimens are examined throughout pregnancy for the presence of antibodies.

After any occasion when fetal cells could have escaped into the maternal circulation (e.g. after threatened abortion, antepartum haemorrhage or cephalic version), Kleihauer's test should be performed immediately to detect fetal cells in the maternal serum.

At delivery, a sample of cord blood is taken to be examined

for the presence of maternal antibodies (Coombs' test) and the haemoglobin and serum bilirubin levels estimated.

Postnatally, if the infant is affected, haemoglobin estimations are carried out daily to check that transfusion is not necessary.

Treatment Antenatally, if levels of antibodies in the maternal blood are high, an early induction of labour may be indicated to prevent severe haemolysis.

After delivery, the cord is left long and untreated, in case an exchange transfusion is necessary via the umbilical vein. The decision as to whether or not transfusion is necessary depends on the haemoglobin estimation.

Exchange transfusion is carried out using Group O Rhesus-negative blood, which washes out much of the bilirubin and antibodies, leaving blood which cannot be haemolysed. By the time the baby has manufactured new blood, most of the antibodies have been destroyed. A single transfusion is usually adequate but occasionally two or even three have to be given. All affected babies should be followed up for some months, as anaemia may develop later.

Prophylaxis The incidence of Rhesus isoimmunization is very much reduced since the development of anti-D. This is a simple intramuscular injection which prevents formation of antibodies if given promptly.

Anti-D is not always necessary for Rhesus-negative mothers, but when it is indicated it must be given within 72 hours of fetal cells entering the maternal blood: that is, before the mother has had time to manufacture antibodies.

Congenital malformations

Congenital malformations may be relatively minor such as extra digits, extra ear lobes, slight webbing of toes or fingers, or major conditions such as the absence of a limb or organ, incomplete canalization somewhere in the alimentary tract, severe heart lesions or genetic disorder.

The medical staff will talk to both parents about the malformation, and suggest to them any treatment necessary and explain the prognosis. The nurse is there to support and comfort the mother during this time, and she must remember that however slight the abnormality the mother will be distressed and worried. Even if the student feels unable to give specific advice, she can give the address of an association which will offer support to the mother.

Infection

The newborn are subject to infection for several reasons. They have left a sterile environment, are in contact with organisms for the first time and their defence mechanisms are immature. Septic spots, infection of the mucous membranes and cord stump are not uncommon, and infections of the respiratory and urinary tracts or bowel may occur. It must be remembered that the mildest complaint may rapidly prove fatal in the newborn.

Infection may be minimized if simple rules of hygiene are observed. The hands should be washed before handling the baby and after changing napkins. All soiled material should be removed from the nursery as soon as possible. Every baby should have individual equipment. All milk-room utensils for preparing and giving feeds should be sterilized.

Cold syndrome

Hypothermia occurs when the temperature falls below 28°C (82°F) and may have serious consequences. Unfortunately, the baby tends to look red and rosy, which is often mistaken as a sign of good health. The skin is cold to the touch and is solid with oedema.

Prevention of cold syndrome is important because all

babies may become chilled if not kept in a reasonably warm atmosphere. In the winter, some form of heating is needed in the bedroom at night, about which the mother should be advised before she leaves hospital.

If hypothermia occurs, the baby must be warmed gradually; if a diagnosis is made, treatment is usually successful.

Sore buttocks

Buttocks may become sore for many reasons. Common causes are inadequate washing and drying of the skin, infrequent changing of napkins, loose stools, rough napkins washed in harsh powders and not adequately rinsed, and candidiasis (thrush).

Frequent changing of napkins, thorough cleansing of the buttocks with soap and water, careful drying and the application of protective baby cream should be effective prevention. However, in *Candida* infection with loose stools, treatment of the underlying condition must be initiated. Midwives vary in their advice for sore buttocks.

Thrush

Thrush is a superficial infection of the mucous membrane of the mouth and alimentary tract caused by the *Candida albicans* (*Monilia albicans*). Infection in the mother may be transmitted to the fetus as he passes through the maternal vagina. On the fourth day after birth the baby is sometimes reluctant to feed and on inspecting the mouth raised greyish white patches, surrounded by an area of inflammation, are found on the inside of the cheeks, the gums and the tongue. The patches resemble milk curd but when gently wiped they cannot be removed (see also page 269).

Treatment Nystatin mixture or nystatin in honey 100 000 units (in 1 ml) is given four times a day for four to seven days. This is usually preferred to gentian violet 1%, because the latter stains the clothing and bed linen and the colour of the baby's lips often frightens the mother.

Care must be taken in the disposal of napkins and the sterilizing of feeding utensils, as thrush can be transmitted from one baby to another by improperly washed hands and contaminated utensils.

Injury

The newborn may sustain an injury during birth or afterwards. Unnecessary pressure on a limb may cause a paralysis or fracture, too rapid delivery of the head might cause intracranial damage, and after birth rough handling may cause bruising, fractures or other injuries. If a nurse suspects the baby has an injury, it must be reported at once, so that appropriate treatment can be initiated.

FURTHER READING

KELNAR, C.J.H. & HARVEY, D. (1981) *The Sick Newborn Baby*. London: Baillière Tindall.

14 Some Social Aspects of Obstetrics

The history of obstetrics is as old as the history of mankind, but only in recent years has there been any form of registration of midwives in Britain. Midwifery began to emerge as a profession in 1881 when the Midwives Institute was established in an attempt to gain recognition of midwives. It was only in 1902 that the *Midwives Act* made registration compulsory, and also empowered the setting up of the Central Midwives Board. Other European countries had state registration of midwives much earlier.

The United Kingdom Central Council

The Central Midwives Board has been the statutory body concerned with the training and practice of midwives, and was set up for the protection of the public. It conducts examinations and keeps a roll of successful candidates. The length of training is at present 18 months for state registered nurses. Every practising midwife has to notify her local Health Authority each year of her intention to continue in practice.

A new regulation in 1955 made it compulsory for every practising midwife to attend a refresher course once in five years. The practising midwife is a practitioner in her own right who is qualified to administer inhalation analgesics and, if necessary, certain drugs.

As a result of the *Nurses, Midwives and Health Visitors Act, 1979*, a new integrated form of control over professional conduct and education for the whole nursing profession has been set up. During 1983 the United Kingdom Central

Council and the four National Boards will take over the functions of existing statutory bodies, including the Central Midwives Board. The organization of a single professional register for all nurses, midwives and health visitors has been proposed, modelled on the Roll of the Central Midwives Board.

The Royal College of Midwives

The Midwives Institute became the College of Midwives in 1941 and in 1947 was granted a royal title. The College is a professional and educational organization for midwives; it exists to ensure the wider education and efficiency of the midwife and to seek to improve her salary and conditions of service.

It is the information centre for the general public on matters pertaining to the profession, and it assists midwives visiting this country from other parts of the world.

NATIONAL HEALTH SERVICE

Since a major reorganization in 1974, the National Health Service has provided health care both in hospital and the community. Until 1982 it was a three-tier structure with overall control by the Department of Health and Social Security in England. However, the 1980 *Health Services Act* effectively removed the Area Health Authorities, creating a two-tier system with the aim of giving greater control at a local level by the new District Health Authorities.

The change in the organization is shown diagrammatically in Fig. 14.1.

In *Scotland* the structure is slightly different and re-organization is still being discussed. At present there is a two-tier system headed by the Scottish Home and Health Department, with 15 Area Health Boards, each of which is divided into Districts.

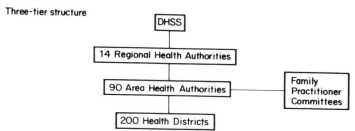

1974 NHS
Three-tier structure

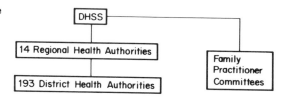

1982 NHS
Two-tier structure

Fig. 14.1 Structure of the NHS, 1974 and 1982.

Department of Health and Social Security (DHSS)

The DHSS has the overall responsibility for the integrated health services, through the Secretary of State for Social Services.

Scotland has its own Scottish Home and Health Department, and a Minister of Health and Social Work.

Regional Health Authority

The Regional Health Authority consists of a salaried chairman and members working on a voluntary basis. It receives guidelines on planning and spending from the DHSS and must ensure that the District Health Authority keeps within agreed costs, and plans the local service within the context of national and regional plans.

The day-to-day management and monitoring of this service is carried out by a salaried team of officers. Each Regional team of officers includes the Medical Officer, Nursing Officer, Finance Officer, Administrator and Works Officer.

There are 14 Regional Health Authorities, each of which is divided into districts with District Health Authorities.

District Health Authority

The District Health Authority serves a small section of the population, mostly between 150 000 and 500 000, and should reflect local needs and responsibilities. The District Health Authority has great freedom in planning and implementing the patterns of health care locally.

The chairman of the District Health Authority is appointed by the Secretary of State, and the remainder of the members should consist of the following people:

1 nurse/midwife/health visitor
1 hospital consultant
1 general medical practitioner
1 university nominee
1 trade union representative
4 local authority representatives
6 members appointed by the DHSS

Each District Health Authority has a District team of professional officers, similar to the Regional team, to advise the Authority on policy and devise means of implementing its decisions. The district thus forms its own units of management with a unit administrator and unit nursing officer, and other officers as they decide. The district maternity services may be organized as one unit, linking both hospital and community care, if the District Health Authority wishes.

The Family Practitioner Committee

General medical practitioners are not employees of the National Health Service, but independently contract their services. Their contracts are administered by Family Practitioner Committees, with separate funding by the DHSS. The former Area Health Authorities were linked to Family Practitioner Committees, but at present each Family Practitioner Committee may work with several District Health Authorities.

Community Health Councils

Linked to each District Health Authority is a Community Health Council, with members nominated by local government district councils, local voluntary bodies and the Regional Health Authority. The function of the Community Health Council is to represent the consumer, by communicating to District Health Authorities their views on local health care provision, and in effect to carry out a 'watchdog' role on behalf of the community.

Provision of maternity services

Since 1948, maternity care has been available free to every pregnant woman, including the provision of midwives and medical staff.

Hospital care Hospital care is available to all patients in the United Kingdom. In some areas there are Consultant Obstetric Units, which are equipped to give more intensive care to patients, such as patients with previous difficult obstetric history, those with medical conditions or elderly primigravidae. The care of a patient is often shared between the hospital and the general practitioner.

General Practitioner Units (GP Units) These are units where the general practitioner who has specialized in obstetrics undertakes the obstetric care in place of a hospital consultant. A community midwife works alongside each general practitioner and usually establishes a relationship of trust with her patients as she cares for them throughout pregnancy and the puerperium. The delivery takes place in the GP Unit, staffed by permanent staff or community staff on rotation.

Domino scheme The domino scheme allows a community midwife, working with the general practitioner, to care for her own patients throughout pregnancy, labour and the puerperium. During labour itself she escorts the patient to hospital, to deliver her there. This scheme permits a delivery within the safe environment of hospital but avoids the more impersonal nature of hospital when the patient does not know the hospital staff. The patient's length of stay in hospital may be as little as six hours.

Home confinement There have been fewer home confinements in recent years, but they are usually permitted at the patient's request when she is healthy, has had at least one previous normal delivery, when there are no problems in her present pregnancy and she has a clean house with adequate heating and help at home. The community midwife and general practitioner usually undertake her care throughout pregnancy, labour and the puerperium.

Many patients consider their own homes to be the most pleasant places for confinement, even if not the safest places.

Emergency Obstetric Service This is a team of hospital staff from a large maternity unit, consisting of a consultant or registrar, anaesthetist, and midwifery sister. They deal with obstetric emergencies, in the home or in small units where there is no obstetric service, for example haemorrhage, abortion or eclampsia.

LOCAL GOVERNMENT

The administration of local government in England since 1974 has been at two levels: county council and district council. The 39 county councils, covering most of England and made up of elected councillors, are responsible for a number of major services including personal social services, education, town and country planning, and police and fire services.

Beneath these, the separately elected district councils have responsibility for housing, local amenities, environmental health and certain other services.

In *Scotland*, the two levels are termed the regional council and district council.

In six densely populated regions of England, local government is administered by metropolitan county and metropolitan district councils (these are Greater Manchester, West Midlands, Merseyside, South Yorkshire, West Yorkshire and Tyne and Wear). In London, there is a different system again, with 33 borough councils which are separate from the Greater London Council.

Each local authority, both at district and county level, carries out its work through specific committees, each related to its own special functions. There is usually a department of permanent staff linked to each committee headed by a chief officer, for example Director of Education, or Director of Social Services.

Personal Social Services

The Personal Social Services are the responsibility of local government Social Service Departments. Their role is to provide a wide range of help, social care and support in the community for individuals or groups in need. The type of help given includes residential homes for the elderly, home help services, domiciliary aids and adaptations for the handicapped, and protective care for neglected or deprived children. Social Service departments have various statutory responsibilities of intervention in the fields of mental illness and child abuse.

Although most social workers are based in the community working in local area teams, some work in hospitals, providing advice and help for patients and their families.

Maternity benefits

Maternity benefits are administered by the local offices of the Department of Health and Social Security, from which application forms are available. Payment is always made through the Post Office.

Maternity Grant This is a lump sum of £25 for each child born, paid to the mother during pregnancy or within three months of delivery, provided that she has been in Britain for more than 26 weeks in the 52 weeks before her expected date of confinement.

Maternity Allowance If the mother has paid the appropriate amount of National Insurance contributions in the relevant tax year, she is eligible for a weekly allowance of £27.25 for 18 weeks, beginning not earlier than 11 weeks before the expected date of confinement.

Maternity Pay Women have the right to remain at work until the 29th week of gestation, and to return to their jobs within 29 weeks of the birth, provided that they have been employed full-time by the same employer for at least two years. They are entitled to take *maternity leave*, during which period they are paid a proportion of their basic salary.

Other benefits related to obstetrics

Prescription and dental charges Women are entitled to free medicines and dental care during pregnancy and for one year after the birth. All children are exempt from prescription charges until they leave school.

Free milk and vitamins All expectant mothers who are receiving Supplementary Benefit, Family Income Supplement, or who have a very low income, are entitled to free milk and vitamins. Milk and vitamin tokens continue to be provided for the child after birth until school age.

Travelling expenses The cost of travel to antenatal clinics can be refunded if the family income is below a certain level.

Child Benefit Child Benefit is payable to all mothers for each child in the family. At present it amounts to £6.85 per week, although it is paid monthly, except in special circumstances.

Single parents A special benefit of £4.25 weekly is available to single parents for the first child, although it is deducted from Supplementary Benefit if this is being paid.

A variety of organizations provide advice and information, and they act as pressure groups for single parents whether they are unmarried, separated, divorced or widowed. One such organization is the National Council for One-Parent Families, a long-established body which presses for improved benefits for one-parent families. Another group, Gingerbread, is a self-help organization with a network of local groups providing help and support for lone parents.

Home helps Home helps may be requested by the hospital or the mother and should be provided by the Social Services

Department, to enable a patient to rest more at home, for example if she has pre-eclampsia. The charge is made according to the family income.

Child Health Clinics

Each local Health Authority runs Child Health Clinics, at which a medical officer is in attendance and health visitors offer advice and help on child care and development. Immunizations are given and routine health checks are carried out.

Baby milk, vitamin drops and fruit juice are sold at subsidized prices. Milk and vitamin tokens can also be exchanged here.

Mortality rates

These are useful indicators of the quality of maternal and child health in the population. The Registrar General publishes a report each year, which includes maternal and infant mortality rates.

There has been a dramatic decrease in maternal and infant mortality since the turn of the century, influenced by a number of factors such as improved diet and living standards, better antenatal and obstetric care, staff training and drug therapy such as antibiotics. However, Britain still lags behind some other countries (Fig. 14.2), notably Sweden whose perinatal mortality rate in 1978 was 9.4 per 1000.

There are also marked variations in mortality rates within the United Kingdom, according to region and social class.

Maternal mortality rate is the number of deaths registered during the year, of women dying from causes attributed to pregnancy and childbirth, per 1000 registered total births per year. The main causes are abortion, pulmonary embolism, eclampsia, ectopic pregnancy, sepsis and haemorrhage.

Perinatal mortality rate is the number of deaths registered during the year of infants in the first week of life, including

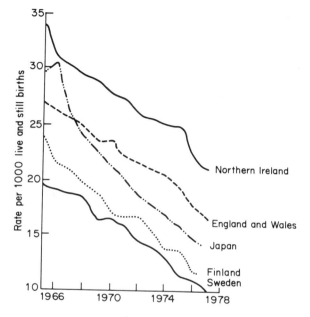

Fig. 14.2 Perinatal mortality since 1965, showing the slow decline in England and Wales compared with other countries.

stillbirths, per 1000 live and stillbirths. This is closely linked to the quality of antenatal care and obstetric practice. The main causes are immaturity, anoxia, intracranial injury, congenital abnormality and social factors.

Neonatal mortality rate is the number of deaths registered during the year, of infants dying under the age of one month (28 days) per 1000 live births. This has not shown the dramatic improvement of the *post-neonatal mortality rate* (death between one month and one year of age). The main causes are respiratory distress syndrome, birth asphyxia, pneumonia, cerebral haemorrhage and congenital malformation.

Infant mortality rate is the number of deaths registered during the year, of infants in the first year of life per 1000 live births. This combines neonatal and post-neonatal rates. The main causes are as for neonatal deaths and accidents (Table 14.1).

Table 14.1. Mortality rates in England and Wales. (Source: Registrar General.)

	1900	1976	1983
Maternal mortality	4.7	0.13	0.09
Infant mortality	146.0	14.2	10.1
Perinatal mortality	Not specified	17.7	10.4
Neonatal mortality	Not specified	9.7	5.9

15 Family Planning: Conception

Family planning means two things: it involves applying a knowledge about conception both to conceive and also to find a suitable method of contraception. Many couples go to special family planning clinics but the nurse may find herself being asked for detailed and sometimes intimate advice by patients either in maternity units (usually about contraception) or in gynaecology departments (usually about conception). The nurse should therefore understand what is involved for conception to occur naturally, how patients can be helped if they have reduced fertility, and how to advise a patient who wants to prevent conception either temporarily or permanently. This chapter discusses conception and infertility, and Chapter 16 deals with contraception.

THE INFERTILE COUPLE

Normally, a couple expect conception to occur whenever they do not take precautions to prevent the spermatozoa from fertilizing the ovum. They do not need to plan coitus on a specific day because with a happy, stable relationship intercourse occurs frequently enough for normal, healthy spermatozoa to survive and reach the ovum.

However, about 10% of married couples find that this is not the case, and the nurse will meet these patients in outpatient clinics. At these clinics each partner will be examined for signs of abnormality or dysfunction which is causing infertility. If nothing is obviously wrong (as is usually the case), then more detailed investigations are carried out:

these are usually done in the outpatient department but some tests require the woman to be an inpatient in the gynaecology ward. Women who have to stay in hospital for investigations are particularly conscious of their apparent inability to conceive and often spend all their day thinking about this.

It is extremely important for the nurse to realize how sensitive her approach must be to these patients. She must help them to feel accepted and relaxed at the clinic, especially on their first visit when they feel so embarrassed. She must ensure privacy, especially when the history is being taken and the couple's very private life is discussed. She must explain why a physical examination is necessary, but understand that many patients find this unpleasant because it turns something normally associated with sexual feelings into something clinical—thus, afterwards, patients may find that the sexual situation too has become a 'clinical' act. Investigations into infertility can even seem to interfere with natural sexual enjoyment. Patients may suppress feelings of embarrassment at a clinic, but they often find that those anxieties reappear in moments of intimacy, causing stress to the marital relationship. For the male partner in particular, investigations into infertility may seem to question his actual virility.

The nurse must therefore understand that psychosexual upsets such as impotence are common in these situations, being manifest especially around the crucial time in the menstrual cycle when the woman is most fertile if intercourse becomes a duty rather than a pleasure. She can show simple yet effective care by listening, by understanding, and by showing that they are not abnormal in experiencing these unwelcome feelings.

Factors which interfere with normal coitus
Some patients experience distressing symptoms which interfere with normal coitus, causing apareunia (complete absence

of intercourse), or dyspareunia (painful or difficult intercourse). Whether of organic or psychogenic origin, the problem is fraught with emotional strain and should be handled very sensitively.

Psychosexual factors have already been alluded to, and are a complex subject which requires specialist skills in psychosexual counselling. Psychogenic dyspareunia is readily differentiated from organic causes by a pelvic examination, but it is often difficult to cure. It may require psychotherapy if the root of the trouble lies, for instance, in childhood or adolescence. Occasionally, simple advice helps to eliminate ignorance and fear, for example the physiotherapist can help by teaching relaxation exercises which reduce tension and relax the levator muscles.

Organic causes may be deep or superficial. Deep dyspareunia is caused by pelvic inflammatory disease, endometriosis and prolapsed ovaries. Superficial dyspareunia is caused by rigid hymen, narrow introitus which may be congenital, poor reconstruction of the perineum following an episiotomy or vaginal repair, or post-menopausal atrophy. Discomfort is also associated with vulvitis and vaginitis, or urethral caruncle. Once the underlying cause has been treated, the dyspareunia is relieved.

Occasionally, physical handicaps are so disabling as to prevent coitus completely. Special guides to assist the physically handicapped are available, for example through the Disabled Living Foundation, but in some cases, artificial insemination using the husband's semen (AIH) may be necessary to achieve a pregnancy.

Examination of patients with infertility

It takes two to make a pregnancy, therefore both partners should always be examined. There are many reasons for infertility in both the male and female and they may need investigating and eliminating systematically in an attempt to find the cause. Current research indicates that in about one-third of couples the husband is sterile, in one-third the wife is sterile, and that in the remaining one-third *sub*fertile group there are factors in both husband and wife. However, it is important not to describe this as either partner's fault because this imparts a burden of guilt, as if the person were actively to blame.

A careful general medical and gynaecological history is taken, together with facts about the duration of infertility, methods of contraception used, frequency of coitus and the patient's awareness of the fertile time in her cycle. This will be followed by a complete medical examination to exclude congenital abnormalities, inflammatory change and other diseases. The husband is also examined thoroughly, noting especially the size and consistency of the testes (both are reduced with poor spermatogenesis), and the presence of the vasa deferenti.

PHYSIOLOGY RELATED TO CONCEPTION

Normally, FSH from the pituitary develops a follicle in the ovary, which then releases the ovum under the influence of LH (see Chapter 2; refer also to Fig. 2.2). This release of the ovum, called ovulation, normally occurs on about day 14 of a menstrual cycle, so this is the woman's most fertile time. Spermatozoa, which were previously deposited in the vagina and have swum up the genital tract, meet the ovum and fertilization takes place (see pages 17–18).

Factors which influence fertility

1. Factors which reduce spermatogenesis. Spermatogenesis can be reduced dramatically but temporarily by transient conditions such as influenza, undue stress or fatigue. Primary spermatogenic failure is one of the commonest reasons for

nale infertility but the cause is still largely unknown. An ncrease in the output of FSH by the pituitary is an attempt to counterbalance this, but usually to little avail. More rarely, permatogenesis may be reduced secondary to orchitis, cryptorchidism, trauma or irradiation. Some chromosomal abnormalities prevent spermatogenesis completely.

2. Factors which cause obstruction. Partial or complete obstruction may be present either in the male, preventing the exit of normal spermatozoa, or in the female, preventing the ovum from reaching or passing down the uterine tube (page 142). In both cases, obstruction can be caused by adhesions following infection (particularly gonorrhoea), or trauma. More rarely, there may be a congenital abnormality which causes obstruction.

3. Factors which reduce motility of spermatozoa. After ejaculation, non-motile spermatozoa cannot reach the ovum o fertilization cannot take place. Sperm motility is adversely affected by pyospermia, or the presence of a varicocele. Abnormal forms do not usually move progressively. Poor cervical mucus (page 192) or sperm–mucus incompatibility inhibits sperm motility.

4. Factors which inhibit ovarian function, causing anovulation (page 192).

5. Uterine abnormalities which may prevent implantation of the ovum. This may be of congenital origin or caused by disease of the endometrium.

INVESTIGATIONS AND TREATMENT

Special investigations may determine various factors affecting fertility. Table 15.1, on pages 190 and 191, summarizes the normal events preceding conception and outlines circumstances under which each investigation would be carried out in order to find the cause of infertility.

Table 15.1 Chart of normal processes preceding conception, showing some factors which cause infertility

Normal	Deviations from normal	Investigations	Possible treatment
Sperms enter vagina at coitus	1. Coitus impossible	History	Psychosexual counselling ?AIH
	2. Non-ejaculation	History ?psychogenic cause ?organic cause	Psychosexual counselling or treat organic cause
	3. No sperms in semen	Semen analysis, then: (a) examine scrotum (?congenital absence of vasa)	None (?AID)
		(b) Serum FSH (?reduced spermatogenesis)	None if severe (?AID)
		(c) Serum karyotype (?abnormal chromosomes)	None (?AID)
		(d) Surgical exploration (?obstruction)	Surgical correction, i.e. vasovasostomy or vaso-epididymostomy
Sperms enter cervical mucus	1. Sperms non-motile at ½ hour	(a) Examine semen for pus cells (b) Examine scrotus for varicocele	Antibiotics if infected Tie varicocele

		Investigation	Treatment
		(b) Examine mucus for: Spinnbarkeit / Ferning / Amount	
Sperms swim up uterine tubes	3. Sperm/mucus incompatible	(a) Sperm penetration test	Clomiphene / Improve mucus or sperm motility
		(b) Post-coital test	Treatment usually unsuccessful in incompatibility
	1. Uterine tubes blocked	Hysterosalpingogram	Tubal surgery, e.g. salpingostomy or salpingolysis
	2. Sperm non-motile at 6 hours	Semen analysis for motility at 6 hours	Discover cause of poor motility (?infection ?varicocele ?unknown)
Fertilization of ovum	No ovum in tube	Test for ovulation (e.g. serum progesterone, day 21) If not ovulating: (a) Serum prolactin (?hyperprolactinaemia)	Bromocriptine if raised
		(b) Serum FSH and LH	Clomiphene if low / No treatment if raised
		(c) Temperature chart (?delayed ovulation)	Clomiphene if delayed ovulation
		(d) Laparoscopic D & C (?pelvic disease, e.g. endometriosis)	Treat disease

Tests for ovulation

After ovulation the ovary produces high levels of progesterone, therefore a test for serum progesterone on about day 21 of the cycle is normally the simplest assessment of ovulation.

Ovulation is also shown, less reliably, by a rise in basal body temperature (Fig. 15.1). A chart of the temperature, taken once daily on waking, should thus have two distinct phases, each of about 14 days, in which the temperature is consistently at least 0.5°C higher from day 14 to day 28 than on days 1 to 14.

The cervical mucus also changes for the few days around ovulation, increasing in amount and showing the Spinnbarkeit phenomenon, which means that it will stretch into a thread of up to 15 cm. When examined microscopically, ovulatory mucus shows a classical 'ferning' pattern (Fig. 15.2).

Histological examination of the endometrium, taken during D and C, should produce evidence of ovulation by showing the secretory changes of the second half of the menstrual cycle. Laparoscopic examination of the ovary at the same time should reveal the corpus luteum on the ovary (see laparoscopic dye test, pages 195–196).

Factors which interfere with ovulation

Undue fatigue and stress (for example, as caused by investigations for infertility) can be sufficient to prevent ovulation. This is one reason why many people become pregnant as soon as they adopt a child and the emotional pressure of childlessness is lifted.

Ovulation is also affected by severe weight loss, or disease such as chronic nephritis, or by endocrine disorders such as diabetes mellitus. Ovulation is restored when the underlying condition is successfully treated.

Insufficient FSH/LH-releasing factor from the hypothalamus will result in anovulation; this is treated with clomiphene which acts through the hypothalamus. The dose

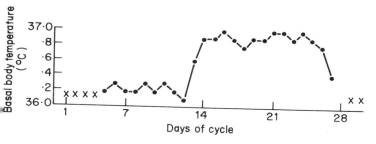

Fig. 15.1 **Temperature chart showing two phases of a normal ovulatory cycle.**

is usually 50–150 mg daily on days 5–9 of the cycle. If the pituitary is normal, this results in increased FSH/LH. If, however, the pituitary does not respond to the releasing factor, as in hypopituitarism, then ovulation can be stimulated using artificial FSH (Pergonal) and LH (Pregnyl). These are potent fertility drugs whose dose must be reassessed every day to prevent multiple ovulation.

Hyperprolactinaemia appears to block the normal release

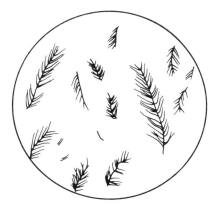

Fig. 15.2 **Diagram showing typical 'ferning' pattern of ovulatory mucus.**

of FSH/LH from the pituitary, but bromocryptine treats this successfully by acting directly on the pituitary. The dose is gradually built up by 2.5 mg twice daily: if this is done too suddenly, nausea, dizziness and Raynaud's phenomenon can occur. (Hyperprolactinaemia occurs normally during breast-feeding and is sometimes, though not always, sufficient to prevent ovulation.)

Patency of uterine tubes

There are three methods of investigating patency of the uterine tubes: hysterosalpingogram, insufflation and the laparoscopic dye test. The first two tests are carried out in the outpatient department and the patient is fully alert during them. The nurse's role is to stay with the patient and comfort her during the discomfort of the procedure. An aperient is necessary the day before the investigations, and if there is any bleeding or inflammation, it should be postponed in order to prevent inflammation being spread to the pelvis.

Hysterosalpingography is carried out in the x-ray depart-ment because it involves the injection of a radio-opaque dye such as iodipamide methylglucamine (Endografin) 70% solution. The dye is introduced via a special cannula, inserted into the uterine cavity after dilatation of the cervical os. The passage of the dye can be observed on the x-ray screen and films can be taken if desired (Figs. 15.3 and 15.4). This test has the advantage of outlining the uterus as well as the tubes, so revealing any abnormalities which may be present such as a bicornuate uterus.

Insufflation is carried out less frequently because it is a less comprehensive test. The procedure is similar to a hysterosalpingogram, but instead of radio-opaque dye, carbon dioxide gas is introduced via the cannula. A manometer measures the pressure of the gas. If the uterine tubes are patent, gas leaks out of them into the peritoneal cavity, causing the manometer pressure to fall. If the tubes are

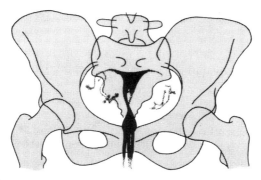

Fig. 15.3 Hysterosalpingography: both tubes patent, radio-opaque dye having escaped into the peritoneal cavity.

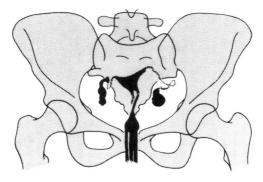

Fig. 15.4 Hysterosalpingography: both tubes blocked at fimbriated ends.

blocked, the pressure will continue to rise. Occasionally, insufflation has the effect of clearing the tube of small amounts of debris.

The *laparoscopic dye test* is carried out in theatre, usually with a general anaesthetic. The patency of the tubes can be demonstrated by observing the passage of dye injected via the cervix: the dye should be seen to spill freely from both tubes.

This test has the advantage that it can be combined with other investigations of infertility, such as the following.

1. Curettings of endometrium can be obtained and sent for histology: if ovulation has occurred, it should show secretory changes.

2. The ovary can be viewed: if ovulation has occurred, the corpus luteum is present.

3. A general pelvic inspection may show signs of disease which interferes with fertility, such as endometriosis, pelvic inflammatory disease, or adhesions from previous inflammation.

The nursing care of a patient having laparoscopy is described on pages 347–348.

Semen analysis

A fresh sample of semen is examined using a microscope. The analysis should be repeated at least once if it is abnormal, since it is affected greatly by temporary factors such as undue fatigue or ill-health. As well as the number of spermatozoa (normally 20–150 million per ml), the motility is also important. Motility is known to be necessary, not only immediately after ejaculation to enter the cervical mucus, but also good motility must be sustained for the spermatozoa to swim up the uterine tubes and then to fertilize the ovum. Large numbers of abnormal forms cause subfertility; at least 50% of spermatozoa should be normal. If the semen is infected, pus cells are present, and this should be treated with antibiotics.

Postcoital test (PCT)

The idea of a PCT is to examine under the microscope a sample of cervical mucus up to ten hours after coitus, to see whether spermatozoa remain motile in the wife's ovulatory mucus. This test should bring to light faulty coital technique or abnormal cervical mucus.

Faulty coital technique is treated by specialist psychosexual counselling and, on the rare occasions when normal coitus may be impossible, artificial insemination using the husband's semen previously obtained at masturbation.

The cervical mucus may be thick and scanty if the sample was taken at the wrong time in relation to ovulation, or if the woman is anovulatory (see tests for ovulation, page 192). Poor quality mucus can be improved with low dose of oestrogens. If chronic cervicitis is thought to be affecting mucus production, this is treated with cervical cautery.

The value of this test is questionable since, within an hour of coitus, most healthy spermatozoa have swum through the cervix and reached the uterus, thus leaving a poor representation for the PCT. Probably of more value is the sperm invasion test.

Sperm invasion test

This test is carried out to assess how well the husband's spermatozoa invade, or penetrate, the wife's mucus. A sample of ovulatory cervical mucus is placed on a glass slide and sent to the laboratory with a fresh specimen of ejaculate. When a drop of ejaculate is placed on the slide, the spermatozoa should be seen actively invading the mucus.

If the spermatozoa do not invade the mucus, it is interesting to compare the effect, firstly of donor semen on the wife's mucus and, secondly, the husband's semen on donor mucus. If donor spermatozoa invade the wife's mucus, this suggests that the mucus is normal and the husband requires further investigation; if the husband's spermatozoa invade the donor mucus, this suggests that the spermatozoa are normal and the wife requires further investigation.

This test should not be confused with extrauterine fertilization. There is no possibility of conception occurring in the laboratory during the sperm invasion test because the ovum is not present in the mucus; it only assesses the activity of sperms in mucus.

ADVICE TO INFERTILE COUPLES

Adoption

When these investigations point to a cause of infertility which has no treatment (see Table 15.1), the couple need to have this explained to them clearly but kindly, so that they can adjust their minds to it. For some who can definitely never be cured (such as those with congenital or chromosomal abnormalities), this news can be a traumatic shock; but for others it may have been expected, especially if they have spent years slowly realizing the situation for themselves.

When the wife is infertile, then the couple may be recommended to apply for adoption, but when the husband is infertile and the wife normal, the couple can choose between adoption and artificial insemination by donor (AID).

Artificial insemination by donor (AID)

This is recommended on medical grounds if the husband is infertile or a carrier of an unacceptable hereditary disease. It is carried out in private and NHS clinics.

The day of ovulation must be assessed as precisely as possible, and insemination should be done on at least two days around the time of ovulation each month. As far as the patient is concerned, the procedure is similar to having a normal smear test, but once the cervix is in view using Cusco's speculum, the donor semen is deposited in the cervical mucus at the os using a syringe. The semen can be fresh or it can have been stored in a liquid nitrogen bank at −196°C.

Artificial insemination by donor is ▮ concept in this country and although it is ▮ creasingly available and successful, there are leg▮ and moral questions which remain unanswered. At p▮ the law states that a child fathered by any man other than t▮ husband is illegitimate, although in fact, many parents do not declare this in order to avoid the unpleasant overtones of a 'bastard' child. There is arguably an element of selecting or controlling our society, by choosing donors who are 'suitable' and rejecting the 'unsuitable' ones. Some people consider that AID is a form of adultery.

Extrauterine fertilization

Very rarely, when the wife has an obstruction of both uterine tubes, an ovum has successfully been removed from the ovary, fertilized with the husband's semen, and then re-implanted into the uterus (a 'test-tube baby'). However, much more work has to be done before this can become more widely available.

FURTHER READING

TSCHUDIN, V. (1982) *Counselling Skills for Nurses*. London: Baillière Tindall.

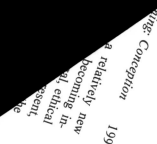

...ethod used by the male or female
p... ...ion at any stage.

In our ... ...ght of every couple, if they so wish, to limit the numbe... ...eir family and to space their children in a way that suits their social and economic needs. Any decisions about birth control should always be taken by the couple themselves, but they often seek advice from the doctor or nurse.

There are many different methods of preventing conception about which the nurse should know, but they must be acceptable to both husband and wife on social, religious and aesthetic grounds. It is not for the doctor or nurse to impose his or her beliefs, but merely to make available the necessary advice.

In the United Kingdom, consultations and contraceptives are provided free of charge to all who ask for them; however, those working in clinics have to bear in mind that sexual intercourse is illegal for children under the age of 16.

The National Health Service (Family Planning) Act of 1967 permits the local authorities to provide family planning facilities. Some have done this by developing new clinics, and others by giving existing Family Planning Association Clinics financial help. General practitioners, obstetricians and hospital departments are also available for advice. The couple can be assured that wherever they go there will be privacy and an opportunity to discuss the method most suited to their needs. Many people still prefer the anonymity of purchasing devices over the counter.

MALE CONTRACEPTION

Condom or sheath

Although these names are often interchanged, a condom is thin and disposable, and a sheath thicker and washable. They are worn over the penis during intercourse to trap the seminal fluid. This method is commonly used because no fitting is necessary; it is reasonably effective although it is unsafe if it is not put on early enough, or if leakage occurs, or if it ruptures. This danger may be lessened by the use of a spermicidal cream.

Coitus interruptus

Coitus interruptus is the withdrawal of the penis from the vagina before ejaculation, and is one of the oldest methods used. The psychological strain placed on both partners is very great and often leads to frustration. The method is wholly dependent on timing and control by the husband and is far from reliable as semen often leaks prior to ejaculation.

FEMALE CONTRACEPTION

Rhythm method (safe period)

The safe period refers to the time in the menstrual cycle when conception cannot take place; that is, away from the time of ovulation. The problem is that the time of ovulation is very difficult to anticipate, but it is easier to assess in retrospect as being 14 days prior to the onset of menstruation each month. If a woman has regular periods, then after keeping a calendar of the exact length of each cycle for 8–12 cycles, she can fairly safely calculate that she will not conceive if she abstains from intercourse for five days on either side of the calculated day of ovulation. This calculation is further substantiated if she also records her basal body temperature every morning for three months: the rise in temperature should occur immediately after the expected day of ovulation (see Chapter 15).

Unfortunately, this method does not allow for irregularities or emotional upsets which may alter the cycle, and it is less reliable at the menopause and during lactation.

Sympto-thermal method

This is a much more reliable adaptation of the rhythm method, used successfully by well-motivated couples who are educated specifically to observe four signs and symptoms of ovulation, and abstain from coitus at this time:

1. dates } as for the rhythm method
2. temperature }
3. cervical mucus—the patient is taught to look for ovulatory mucus (see page 192)
4. pain—some women are aware of a slight pain on one side of the lower abdomen on the day of ovulation.

In recent years women have become increasingly better educated about their own bodily functions, which has resulted in many of them understanding much more about conception and contraception. The World Health Organization has responded to this by expanding knowledge about the sympto-thermal method, which can of course be adapted to help the couple who are trying to conceive.

Occlusive caps

There are several types of cap which cover the cervix and mechanically obstruct the entrance of spermatozoa. They must be fitted by a doctor and need checking for fit at intervals, especially after childbirth or loss of weight.

Diaphragm (dutch cap) A diaphragm is a shallow rubber cap fitting across the vagina from the posterior fornix to the ridge behind the pubic arch. Diaphragms can only be used if

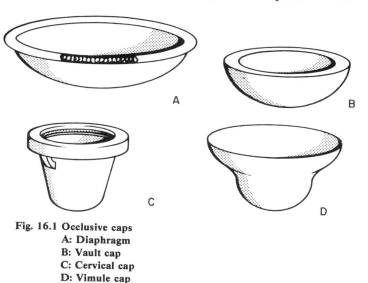

Fig. 16.1 Occlusive caps
    A: Diaphragm
    B: Vault cap
    C: Cervical cap
    D: Vimule cap

the muscle tone of the vagina and perineum is good (Fig. 16.1A).

Vault cap The vault cap is bowl shaped, thin in the centre and thicker at the rim, which clings to the vaginal vault by suction. It is essential that the cervix is short and healthy (Fig. 16.1B).

Cervical cap A cervical cap covers the vaginal portion of the cervix rather like a thimble. It can only be used if the cervix is long and of equal diameter at any level, and if the patient can reach it easily (Fig. 16.1C).

Vimule cap The vimule cap is a combination of the cervical and vault-type cap. It has a domed centre and a flanged rim which adheres to the vault by suction. This is useful when vaginal tone is poor (Fig. 16.1D).

All caps are made in a variety of sizes and must be fitted individually. The patient is taught how to insert, remove and care for them. She is sent home with an imperfect practice cap and asked to return a week later with the cap in position. This serves two purposes, to test the patient's ability to insert the cap and to allow the doctor to check the fit. Nervousness at the first visit often causes vaginismus (spasm in the vagina) and a large enough cap may not be given. At the next visit a perfect cap is supplied together with spermicidal cream which should always be used. The cap should not be removed for at least six hours and preferably longer after intercourse. The patient should be encouraged to get into the habit of inserting the cap regularly, for example every night when she uses the bathroom.

Chemical contraceptives

There are a variety of chemical substances which kill spermatozoa. They are incorporated in jellies, creams, pastes, pessaries and aerosol foams. Instructions vary and they should be studied carefully and the correct amount used. There is quite a high proportion of failure with chemical contraceptives alone, but in conjunction with a cap or sheath they are very effective.

Intrauterine contraceptive devices (IUCDs)

Intrauterine contraceptive devices are small plastic devices which are introduced into the uterine cavity by means of a special applicator (Fig. 16.3). Their exact mode of action is uncertain but a fertilized ovum reaches the uterus before it is sufficiently developed to embed. The copper coils are being used more frequently because the copper itself increases contraceptive action by making the environment unfavourable for implantation.

The designs of IUCD are shown in Fig. 16.2.

The Copper 7 can be used for nulliparous women because

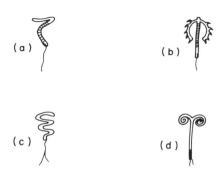

Fig. 16.2 Intrauterine contraceptive devices
    (a): the Copper 7 (Gravigard)
    (b): the Cooper T (Multiload)
    (c): the loop (Lippes loop)
    (d): the double spiral (Saf-T-Coil)

it is so small. Many patients prefer the IUCD because they can forget about taking contraceptive precautions for years. A few women expel the device and this occurs around the time of menstruation within the first six months after insertion: for this reason each patient should be taught to check that it is still in position by feeling for the string at the cervix each month.

Complications Pregnancy occurs in a small number of cases, and the device is often delivered with the placenta. Menstruation is often heavier and prolonged for several cycles but should subside; if it does not, a doctor should be consulted. For this reason the IUCD is contraindicated for women who already have menorrhagia, and also if there are submucus fibroids, cervicitis or suspected malignancy. It is not recommended if there is pelvic inflammatory disease because it can exacerbate pelvic inflammation; nor if there is a history of subfertility because it can cause tubal pregnancy.

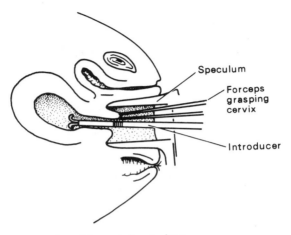

Fig. 16.3 Insertion of intrauterine device.

Oral contraceptives

Most oral contraceptives work by inhibiting ovulation. There are about 30 different brands available with various dosages of each constituent, but these fall into three different categories. As there are different modes of action and slight variations in the number of days on which tablets are taken, it is imperative that the instructions given with each product are followed carefully.

Combined pill This is an oestrogen–progestogen formula, which is the most efficient of all the pills. The oestrogen suppresses ovulation by inhibiting the hypothalamic releasing factors for FSH and LH. As a result, FSH secretion is lowered (so a follicle is not *stimulated*), and the LH peak is abolished (so an ovum is not *released*). The progestogen inhibits proliferation of endometrium (so *implantation* is prevented, should ovulation and fertilization occur). This effect is represented in Fig. 16.4.

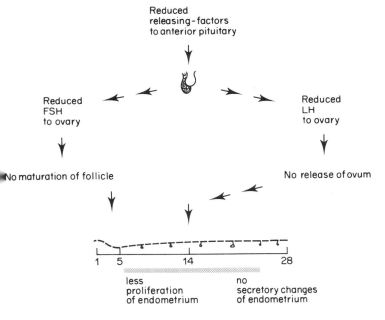

Fig. 16.4 **Effect of the combined pill on the menstrual cycle (compare with Fig. 2.2).**

The combined pill is usually taken for 21 days, from the 5th to the 25th day of the cycle. During the seven days in between each course, no tablets are taken, unless a placebo is given to keep the woman in the habit of remembering her pill. Withdrawal bleeding occurs in this time.

Sequential pill This is a course of two distinct kinds of tablet, usually of a different colour. One contains oestrogen only and is taken for several days, before the other containing progesterone is taken for the remainder of the course. The action of each synthetic hormone is the same as described for the combined pill, but is said to produce a nearly normal physiological effect with a lower total dose of hormone taken. However, it does occasionally allow pregnancy to take place.

Progestogen-only pill (the mini-pill) This consists of progestogen only, therefore the oestrogen effect is excluded altogether, making it less reliable. The progestogen simply alters cervical mucus, making sperm penetration less likely, and diminishes endometrial proliferation, making implantation less likely.

Menstruation does not occur because cyclic changes are depressed; the endometrium is constantly kept minimal and does not shed itself for the duration of pill taking. The progestogen-only pill is therefore taken daily without a break.

Oral contraceptives can have certain side-effects which include weight gain, nausea, breast heaviness and headache, but these tend to diminish in time. More dangerously, the oestrogen content of the pill increases the risk of vascular disease, notably deep vein thrombosis, hypertension and myocardial or cerebral infarction. This risk is increased in women over 35 years of age and by heavy smoking and obesity. The oestrogen-containing pill is also contraindicated with some carcinomas which proliferate under the influence of oestrogen. In diabetes mellitus, stability may be affected and it may be necessary to adjust treatment. For these reasons, women taking oral contraceptives should be seen by a doctor at least once per year to check their weight, blood pressure, and sometimes extra tests such as liver function tests and cervical smear.

Sterilization

Sterilization should always be thought of as a permanent method of birth control once the couple's family is complete; its finality should be explained to husband and wife before they both sign the consent form for operation. However, in practice it is not always final: failures do occur and also patency has successfully been restored after sterilization.

Contrary to many fears, sterilization does not cause loss of libido but rather it usually enhances the sex life because it removes the fear of an unwanted pregnancy.

Either the male or the female partner may be sterilized.

Female sterilization Female sterilization consists simply of causing an interruption in the uterine tube so that spermatozoa cannot reach an ovum which has been released from the ovary. It does not affect ovulation or the woman's normal hormonal cycles, so she continues to menstruate as usual until the menopause. The woman is protected immediately from further pregnancy.

In order to be sterilized, a woman may choose one of two operations.

Laparoscopic application of a clip This can be performed under general or local anaesthetic, involving two tiny cuts in the abdomen. The uterine tubes are both identified and occluded by the application of an inert silicone clip (Fig. 16.5).

This operation causes minimal damage to the tubes and is reversed more simply than a ligation. The woman may be in hospital as a day patient, returning home on the same evening if she had a local anaesthetic and if there were no complications.

Nursing care of a patient having a laparoscopy is given in Chapter 27.

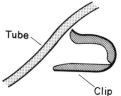

Fig. 16.5 Application of a clip to the uterine tube.

Tubal ligation This operation requires a mini-laparotomy under general anaesthetic, and consists of removing a small wedge-shaped area from each uterine tube. The mid-portion of the tube is usually chosen. The uterine tube and its blood vessels are ligatured, using a non-absorbable suture (Fig. 16.6). Occasionally, the tubes are simply tied, but this is less reliable because recanalization can occur between adjacent portions of the tube, which allows fertilization and pregnancy to ensue.

Male sterilization A vasectomy creates an interruption in the passage of spermatozoa from the testes at ejaculation (Fig. 16.7). It literally means the removal of part of the vasa deferenti, via a small incision in the scrotum. It does not affect the male hormones or prevent ejaculation, but merely causes the seminal fluid which is ejaculated to be free of spermatozoa.

The operation, which is simple to perform, is carried out under local anaesthetic. The patient's greatest need is for reassurance and the nurse must find the most effective way of meeting that need. Grown men do not like to show their need for reassurance but the nurse must realize that the patient is extremely apprehensive, and even though he may be considerably older than herself she should overcome her shyness

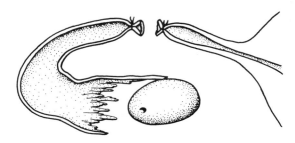

Fig. 16.6 Ligation of the uterine tubes.

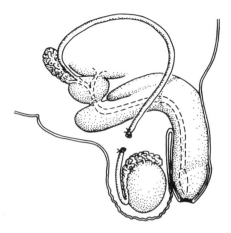

Fig. 16.7 Ligation of vas deferens.

in order to comfort him. She should try to distract him from the operation by involving him in conversation, preferably with *him* talking (he is unable to concentrate on listening).

After the operation the patient may require mild analgesics such as paracetamol. There are usually one or two catgut sutures which will dissolve, and a gauze dressing which may be removed the following day when he takes a bath. The patient should be advised to contact his doctor if he is worried about swelling or bruising of the scrotum, but these complications are rarely severe. A simple scrotal support can often relieve swelling.

Intercourse may be resumed at any time, but other contraceptive precautions must be taken until at least two semen analyses show that no sperms are present. Spermatozoa which persist in the duct system could cause a pregnancy for up to a year after vasectomy.

17 The Menopause

The menopause is the cessation of menstruation brought about by hormonal changes. It normally occurs at the age of 45 to 50 years in British women, although occasionally it is artificially induced in younger women, for example by bilateral oophorectomy.

The menopause is accompanied by general signs and symptoms which many women dread and refer to as the *climacteric*. These symptoms can occur from two to three years before until a year after the cessation of menstruation.

The nurse will meet many gynaecology patients around the time of the menopause, who will be grateful for the professional advice she can give to dispel fears, myths or suspicions. In order to be of help, the nurse must therefore understand the physiological changes which take place.

Physiological changes

As a woman becomes older, the oocytes gradually become unresponsive to FSH stimulation, therefore graafian follicles fail to mature (refer to Chapter 2). The resultant fall in the level of circulating oestrogens causes the pituitary to increase its release of FSH and LH, but despite this increased stimulation the oocytes still do not respond. Eventually ovulation and the menstrual cycle cease completely, and the pituitary ceases to produce high levels of FSH and LH.

Signs and symptoms

Irregular menstruation Menstruation continues while the ovarian cycle is occurring (see Chapter 2), but once the level of oestrogens falls markedly, this cycle ceases. However, the change takes a few years to occur and meantime even small amounts of oestrogen can continue to maintain a proliferative endometrium which breaks down at intervals, giving irregular menstruation.

Menstrual disturbance is one of the signs of malignant disease (see Chapter 24), and unfortunately diagnosis can be delayed if irregular bleeding from carcinoma is confused with menopausal symptoms.

Hot flushes Hot flushes are one of the most unpleasant symptoms brought about by the sudden dilatation of blood vessels supplying the skin. They may be frequent and tend to be worse in hot weather, and in the few days following a period or absent period. They can cause a great deal of embarrassment, especially severe flushes followed by profuse sweating. Hot flushes are the most common indicators for oestrogen therapy.

Psychological changes A woman may find herself experiencing psychological changes which can be very disturbing. Examples of these changes are depression, irritability, lack of concentration, emotional instability, and loss of libido.

To some extent, these symptoms are thought to be caused by the profound psychological impact of realizing that the menopause signifies the end of childbearing years and heralds the beginning of old age. Whatever the cause, women seek understanding and help to maintain their respect for their self image—even if that self image is changing.

Malaise Malaise, or just 'not feeling well', is probably the vaguest of all menopausal symptoms; it is difficult to describe but headaches, mild giddiness and insomnia all lead to fatigue. This is not only tiresome to the woman herself but irritating to those around her.

Post-menopausal symptoms As a result of the lack of oestrogens, various changes occur after the menopause. The vagina becomes dry, its vascularity is reduced and the acidity is lowered to pH 7.2 which encourages infection (Chapter 22). Vulvitis, kraurosis and dyspareunia may occur (Chapter 21). The uterus becomes small and fibrous, and its supportive ligaments become lax which predisposes to prolapse (Chapter 26). There is a progressive decalcification of bones with osteoporosis, and the woman is more prone to arthritis and bony fractures.

Hormone replacement therapy

When signs and symptoms become intolerable, a woman should be advised to consult her doctor, first because hormone replacement therapy has eliminated many of the discomforts associated with the menopause, but also in order to check that they are not signs of other disease.

Treatment is usually by giving oestrogens, either by cream to apply locally, or tablets to give a systemic effect. It is thought that the high levels of FSH and LH cause symptoms, and that these are lessened when circulating oestrogen levels are reduced gradually, not suddenly.

Hormone replacement therapy is also beneficial because it delays the long-term effects of the menopause, such as osteoporosis.

18 Preoperative Care in Major Gynaecological Surgery

Many gynaecological operations are minor, such as dilatation and curettage, or purely investigatory, such as laparoscopy. In this chapter the preoperative care of the patient having a major operation is dealt with—operations such as:

abdominal operations: abdominal hysterectomy, myomectomy, oophorectomy, salpingostomy

vaginal operations: vaginal hysterectomy, the Manchester repair, local and radical vulvectomy.

Admission

The patient is usually admitted to the ward 48 hours before operation in order to ensure that she has a good rest. Nurses can help her at this time by making time to establish a rapport with her in order that she can trust them enough to ask questions, which are often of a very personal nature. This time also enables patients to find a fellow patient who often becomes mutually supportive postoperatively.

The actual admission procedure is of very special importance in the gynaecology unit, so it is essential to afford privacy and time for questions at this stage, even though this is often difficult to arrange. A cup of tea or coffee and a calm orderly atmosphere, regardless of the amount of work being done, are invaluable in establishing the confidence of the patient—and her husband—in the staff and her surroundings.

The husband is often glad to have a chat with 'the professionals' about his wife's operation, because he probably has no other source of accurate information about what will be done and how it will affect both his wife and himself. He will also want to know, with his wife, exactly when the operation is likely to take place, at what times he may visit her, and how long she will be expected to stay. Should his consent for operation be necessary, as for sterilization, it is important to ascertain that he will be visiting again before operation, as this may be difficult if he has small children to care for.

Having been allowed to say goodbye to her husband in privacy, the new patient will be shown the layout of the ward and become acquainted with her neighbours. Her temperature, pulse and respiration are recorded, the patient weighed, and the urine tested for sugar and protein. An identification band bearing her name is fixed to her wrist.

Examination and investigation

A complete general and local examination (see Chapter 20) will be made by the doctor, including the following investigations.

Midstream specimen of urine if urinary infection is suspected. If the vaginal wall is prolapsed, the resultant distortion of the urethra and disturbance of bladder function may predispose to infection.

High vaginal swab if vaginal discharge is present, in order to treat with appropriate antibiotics before the operation.

Cervical smear if this was not done in the outpatient clinic.

Haemoglobin estimation if the patient is suffering from menorrhagia, because her haemoglobin level is likely to be reduced. Desirable levels vary, but most surgeons prefer not to operate with a haemoglobin level less than 10.2 g per 100 ml. Should transfusion be required, and time permits, it is advisable for the operation to be postponed as the risk of thrombotic emboli is thought to be reduced when there is an interval of a week or so between transfusion and operation.

Blood group and cross-matching to prepare for transfusion in theatre should this become necessary.

Chest x-ray if there is any doubt about the patient's fitness for anaesthetic.

Explanations and consent

Consent for operation should not be obtained until examination and investigations have been completed and the full implications of the operation have been explained. Although consent is the responsibility of the medical staff, the nurse may often find she needs to reinforce the doctor's words, because patients are often shy of questioning the medical staff (Fig. 18.1). She must therefore ensure that for each patient her explanations are correct. For example, two patients in the same ward may think they are having the same operation—'hysterectomy'—but this may not be so. One may have a vaginal wound, and the other an abdominal one; one will wake up with a pack and catheter in situ, the other will not; the operation may or may not be accompanied by bilateral oophorectomy, consequently the hormone profiles may remain totally unchanged or become radically different. The nurse must therefore find out *exactly* what is to be done at operation, so that she can tell the patient these details.

Physiotherapy

Physiotherapy has an important role to play in both the pre- and post-operation period.

Breathing exercises and leg movement should be taught to each patient individually by the nurse or physiotherapist so that the patient may be familiar with their use immediately after waking from the anaesthetic. In cases of genital prolapse it is of special importance because:

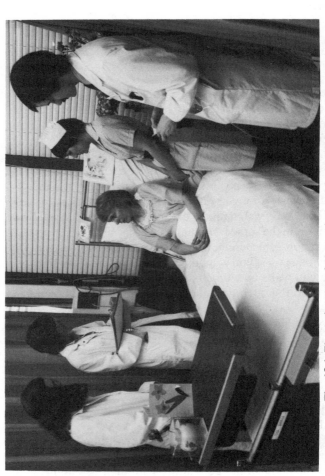

Fig. 18.1 The patient can feel very isolated in hospital, even when

1. the tone of weakened pelvis floor muscles can be improved by exercise
2. chronic bronchitis or excessive obesity may have been contributing factors to the original prolapse.

If there is stress incontinence, the patient may need some encouragement to breathe deeply as sometimes this provokes coughing, and the long association of leaking urine whilst coughing will inhibit her from deliberately taking any such risk.

Smoking is discouraged, and if a cough is present inhalations such as of compound tincture of benzoin (5 ml diluted in 600 ml of water) may be helpful in loosening secretions or as a prophylactic measure.

Where possible, all patients are encouraged to be mobile in between periods of thorough rest and relaxation before the operation.

Diet

Adequate hydration preoperatively is believed to help in the prevention of postoperative thrombosis and shock, therefore the patient is encouraged to drink at least 2 litres of fluid in 24 hours. The diet may be supplemented by vitamin C in the form of ascorbic acid, 50 mg three times a day, as this improves the health of tissue and promotes healing. If there is a deficiency of iron, ferrous sulphate or some similar preparation may be given by mouth.

Patients having abdominal operations may eat a full diet. For vaginal operations a low-residue diet is often given for 48 hours preoperatively because a completely empty bowel is especially important when surgery is contemplated on the posterior vaginal wall.

Drugs

Oestrogen therapy may be given to patients undergoing vaginal surgery who have reached the menopause, because the withdrawal of oestrogens often results in a decrease of lactobacillus, which in turn predisposes to vaginitis. In this case, small doses of oestrogen such as ethinyl oestradiol 0.01 mg orally per day for one week, and oestroform pessaries 0.5 mg at night may be used.

Antibiotics may be given orally if there is infection of the genital tract, and if treatment with sulphadimidine and stilboestrol pessaries applied locally is considered insufficient. Occasionally, the operation may be postponed until the cervix and surrounding tissues are clean and healthy. Intravenous antibiotics may be indicated in cases of severe peritonitis prior to a laparotomy.

Vitamin or iron supplements—see 'Diet'.

Hypnotics are usually prescribed to ensure a good night's sleep before the day of operation. However, their use must be backed by good nursing such as maintaining a happy, peaceful atmosphere in the ward, answering any little worries, and giving a warm drink at bedtime.

Hygiene and shaving

A bath is given at least daily from admission, and a bactericidal soap such as hexachlorophene may be used. Special attention is paid to cleaning the umbilicus prior to abdominal surgery.

The pubic hair is removed by shaving whenever the surgeon requests this. Any of four types of shave may be desired.

1. Abdominal shave.
2. Vulval shave.
3. Perineal shave.
4. Complete shave.

Soap and water or talcum powder may be used when shaving the pubic hair. The patient is placed in the dorsal position for abdominal or vulval shaving, and turned to the left lateral position for the perineal and anal area.

Shaving always causes an embarrassing itch as the hair regrows, therefore the nurse need not shave the total area if only a partial shave is necessary. When a close shave is not desired, the hair may be clipped using scissors or barber's clippers.

Preparation of the bowel

The nature and timing of the preoperative aperient vary with the surgeon's wishes. Any of the following may be used.

1. Sennokot or cascara compound 2 tablets, 36 hours previously.
2. Suppositories such as bisacodyl (Dulcolax) or a simple enema if indicated.
3. Occasionally, a retention enema of warm olive oil (150 ml) introduced slowly into the rectum in the evening, to be followed the next morning by a soap and water enema.

Special note. *Never* should the number of patients who are given an enema or suppositories exceed the number of lavatories in the ward. This thoughtless practice causes immense anxiety to patients. Careful planning and liaison between nurses is called for when there are large numbers of patients to prepare for theatre.

Although an empty bowel is important, especially for vaginal surgery, too vigorous purgation is thought by some to be one of the causes of the abdominal distension usually apparent on the third or fourth postoperative day.

Preparation of the vagina by douche

Vaginal douche is performed at times other than prior to surgery, but it is described here because of its supposed value

in increasing acidity and thereby decreasing susceptibility to
infection before an operation. It is particularly helpful as
prophylaxis for a patient who has had previous infection, or
one who has reached the menopause and whose vagina is
deficient in bactericidal activity.

Requirements
    Douche or bedpan
    Disposable gloves
    Warmed antiseptic lotion
    Wool swabs
    Douche can, tubing, douche nozzle or straight catheter
size 8EG, 16FG, tapered connection, clamp
    1-litre jug of lotion at 41°C
    Vulval pad
    Disposal bags, for soiled dressing and instruments

Lotions Douches are only given when prescribed, therefore
the solution to be used is the doctor's decision. Common
lotions used are:
    water
    normal saline
    bicarbonate of soda 1 : 160 (1 teaspoonful in 500 ml)
    proflavine 1 : 2000
    lactic acid 0.5% or 1%; or vinegar 1 : 160—for treatment
of senile vaginitis

Procedure The nurse should explain to the patient what
she is going to do, and why, and assure her that this is
soothing rather than uncomfortable in any way. Whilst the
patient then empties her bladder, the nurse can assemble her
equipment.
    The patient is placed on the bedpan in the dorsal position
and covered with a loose sheet or blanket. She may be asked
to lift the blanket to expose the vulva when the nurse returns
from washing her hands.

The vulva is swabbed using the warmed antiseptic lotion, as described on page 248. The nurse picks up the catheter with the right hand, allows some of the lotion to run into the bedpan and clamps off the catheter once the tubing is free of air. If this is allowed to run over the thigh, the patient will know that the temperature is comfortable.

Keeping the labia separated with the left hand, the nurse gently introduces the catheter into the vagina in a backward direction for about 8 cm. The clamp is released and the lotion allowed to run into the vagina fairly slowly. During irrigation the catheter may be rotated slowly to allow thorough cleansing of the parts.

When all the lotion has run through, the catheter is withdrawn. The patient is assisted into the sitting position and asked to cough or strain (if there is no wound); this encourages the remaining fluid to drain. She then lies back again and the vulva is thoroughly dried with swabs. The bedpan is removed and the patient is asked to turn on to her left side so that the perineum and buttocks can be dried. A fresh vulval paid is applied and the patient left warm and comfortable.

Preparation of the vagina by painting

Sometimes painting of the vagina is thought preferable to a douche. There are other indications for painting, notably the treatment of *Candida albicans*.

Requirements

Bowl of warm lotion

Dry swabs and vulval pad

Gallipot of paint, e.g. aqueous solution of gentian violet 1 %

Sim's speculum and sponge-holding forceps with gauze-covered swab

Paper towel

Good light or torch

Procedure The patient is prepared as for a douche, but she should adopt the Sim's position. After swabbing the vulva the lubricated speculum is inserted using the right hand, and is then held with the left so that the right hand is then free to grasp the sponge holder. The swab is dipped into the paint and inserted into the vagina. Painting begins at the vault and works downwards. Care must be taken to paint the whole vagina; this is easier when a coloured paint is being used. A vulval pad is secured with a T-bandage and the patient warned if the solution is likely to stain her clothing.

The morning of operation

Depending on the time of operation and the anaesthetist' preference, food may be withheld from 12 midnight or a light breakfast of tea and toast given. Most anaesthetists agree that food should be withheld for a minimum of six hours and fluid for five hours preoperatively.

The patient is dressed in an operation gown and socks, dentures and hair grips are removed, and the wedding ring covered with adhesive plaster. The hair is tied back from the face and lipstick and coloured nail varnish removed. The bladder is emptied at the time the premedication is given and the vulval pad changed but not fastened. All details are recorded on the anaesthetic form and the patient's identification checked by the ward sister, this is either written on the patient's skin with a skin pencil or some type of wrist label. It is essential to see that all reports of investigations, x-rays, old and current notes are ready with the anaesthetic instrument to accompany the patient to the theatre. The nurse will find a busy operating list is likely to run more smoothly if a small list is compiled for each patient the night before, which enables each item to be ticked as it is checked.

FURTHER READING

FISH, E.J. (1979) *Surgical Nursing*, 10th ed., Chapter 6. London: Baillièr Tindall.

19 Postoperative Care in Major Gynaecological Surgery

The postoperative days provide the nurse with ample opportunity to give patients good nursing care, with physical, psychological and emotional support. The first hours in particular allow her to convey care by the valuable form of communication—touch. Even though anaesthetics and heavy sedation cause amnesia, many patients who felt fragile after their operation recall feeling well looked after when nursing procedures have been carried out gently and soothingly.

The lists of patients for gynaecological theatre tend to be very long, which makes the nurse's duty to treat each patient as an individual particularly difficult. However, the nurse must constantly guard against the temptation to treat any patient as 'yet another D & C', by drawing alongside each one as a fellow-human who is dependent on nurses for special care.

Immediate care and observations

The nurse who receives the patient from theatre needs to ascertain certain information from the theatre or recovery room nurse, to satisfy herself that she knows the exact condition of the patient for whom she is caring. Indeed, without this knowledge she is blindly taking responsibility for a patient who needs thorough and specific care.

Information to ask for
1. Name of the patient.
2. Nature of the operation.
3. Drugs which have been given (ensure that these were *signed* for).
4. Particular problems encountered or any complication to be looked for.
5. When oral feeding can recommence.

Observations to make with the theatre nurse
1. Blood loss: on wound dressing and/or on vulval pad.
2. Catheter or drainage tubes.
3. Intravenous infusion: rate of flow, site of needle.
4. Vaginal pack.

In the ward the patient is received into a clean bed and placed in the left lateral position, the nurse taking care to see that the airway is not obstructed at any time.

The following *additional observations* are now recorded.
5. Skin—colour and feel. Note cyanosis, pallor, or clamminess.
6. Respiration—rate. Note gurgling sounds which indicate early obstruction of airway.
7. Pulse—volume, rate. Note tachycardia or poor volume.
8. Temperature—of axilla. Note pyrexia; prevent coldness.
9. Blood pressure—note gradual or sudden fall in pressure.

These observations, combined with those listed above, will be repeated and recorded at frequent intervals, and at least half-hourly until they are stable within normal limits.

Care of the patient's general well-being

Once the patient shows signs of rejecting the airway and it is finally removed, she may be given a pillow; after this it is unnecessary for the nurse to stay at the bedside, but she should observe the patient frequently. An intramuscular narcotic such as papaveretum 20 mg may be given four-hourly to alleviate pain and promote a sense of well-being. This may be accompanied by perphenazine 5 mg or a similar drug to allay postoperative vomiting. When the drugs have had time to take effect, the patient's face and hands may be washed, her own nightgown put on and her mouth rinsed. If she is not feeling nauseated, sips of water are welcome at this stage.

The patient should be encouraged to move her legs every hour in bed, and to continue with her breathing exercises. She must also be informed about the operation as soon as she is sufficiently alert. This will need to be repeated on more than one occasion as a certain amount of amnesia is associated with anaesthetics and the regular use of narcotics.

Local care

The vulval pad should be observed and replaced with a sterile one as necessary. Any heavy loss is recorded on the chart, and if severe the doctor should be informed (see 'Haemorrhage', page 236).

Abdominal operations are usually performed through a transverse Pfannenstiel incision, although occasionally a midline incision is used for exploratory operations. The Pfannenstiel allows for greater movement postoperatively and the indefinable scar at the pubic hairline is invisible even with a mere bikini (hence its nickname, the 'bikini-cut').

Care of the bladder

Special care of the bladder is vital after gynaecological surgery, because of the close proximity of the urethra (in vaginal operations) or the ureters and the bladder itself (in abdominal operations). A fluid intake and output chart must always be kept accurately in order to check that the urinary system is resuming its normal function.

If there is no indwelling catheter, as after most abdominal

operations, micturition is usually re-established within 12 to 16 hours. Accuracy in measurement and recording of fluid balance is vital in order for the nurse to assess at a glance at the chart whether the patient is passing urine normally, or if there is retention, or retention with overflow (see 'Urinary complications', page 237).

If there is an indwelling catheter, as in most vaginal operations involving the anterior vaginal wall, management will depend upon the surgeon's wishes. Usually the bladder is drained continuously, thus preventing distension and strain on the new suture line. Clear urine should begin to drain shortly after the patient returns to the ward; this must be checked frequently because kinking of the catheter or tubing causes back pressure and harmful distension, as well as intense discomfort.

The morning after operation

By the morning after the operation the patient should be in the upright position supported by pillows. Pressure on the perineum can be relieved, after vaginal surgery, by inclining her to one side on a sorbo ring or square of foam rubber. At some time during the first 24 hours she will be assisted out of bed to use the commode and helped to walk a few steps. She will probably enjoy some tea and toast at breakfast time, although this should be withheld if there is vomiting or if bowel sounds are not beginning to re-establish themselves.

During the day, a bed bath should be given and pressure areas attended to; the hair should be brushed and combed, the teeth cleaned and the bed made as necessary.

A vulval toilet should be performed to help the patient to feel fresh despite the slight vaginal loss. Once the patient has regained strength she can use a bidet (page 125) but at this early stage she will appreciate having the area swabbed with an antiseptic solution such as cetrimide 0.1% or Savlon 1 in 100. Each swab is used once only, working from above downwards and from the labia majora inwards to the labia minora and vestibule. Gloves or forceps may be used.

CARE AFTER THE FIRST 24 HOURS

Analgesics
The injections of the first 24 hours will now gradually be replaced by oral analgesics such as paracetamol 1 g four-hourly. The speed at which this is achieved will vary from patient to patient. It is thought that the need for strong analgesics is lessened when nurses discuss postoperative pain and its relief with the patient before she goes to theatre; also that in the long run fewer injections are required if sufficient have been given in the early postoperation period. The nurse, however, must not withhold relief on the assumption that care and foresight have already been applied in this way: unfortunately, many patients are denied comfort through this misapprehension. The nurse must use her skill and discretion in assessing the degree of pain and evaluating with the patient the appropriate treatment to meet that need. Intelligent anticipation of the patient's needs will prevent the pain becoming too severe to be treated by milder analgesics, and will also add to the patient's feeling of security. Most patients will not ask until the pain becomes unbearable.

Analgesics offered and given willingly and caringly are much more effective than when given resentfully or even just 'routinely'.

Diet
Small helpings of a light diet will be given. After abdominal surgery this will gradually be increased to a full diet rich in protein by about the fourth day. After vaginal surgery the diet may be low in residue for the first three to four days, and a full diet resumed once there has been a normal bowel action.

Vitamin C will be resumed to aid the healing of tissues. The fluid intake should be at least 3 litres in 24 hours; this is especially important if there is an indwelling catheter.

Physiotherapy

Leg movements and deep breathing exercises will be continued. The patient should be reminded not to lie with her legs crossed or knees bent for prolonged periods, and that sitting upright assists lung expansion. She will be out of bed for longer intervals each day, and after a few days she will probably be sitting at the table for all meals. Continuous bladder drainage need in no way prevent her getting up and about, and the plastic drainage bag can be pinned unobtrusively inside her dressing-gown; care must be taken to prevent urine siphoning back by keeping the bag below the level of the bladder. Alternatively, the catheter may be spigoted and released at intervals.

This is a particularly good time to teach pelvic floor exercises, partly because they are especially helpful at this time, and partly because the patient is very receptive to learning about anything which will aid her recovery. However, they should be taught by a physiotherapist who will gradually increase the exercises from a very gentle beginning so as to avoid harmful strain to muscles which have been cut. Adequate amounts and careful timing of analgesics will enable the patient to cooperate well in this.

Care of the bowel

During anaesthesia, peristalsis is reduced with a subsequent delay in the passage of faeces: this in part accounts for the abdominal distension which occurs before normal peristalsis is resumed.

Patients become apprehensive about the first bowel action because they anticipate causing strain on the sutures. The nurse must therefore give explanations, even to patients who do not voice their fear, and carry out any treatment with understanding.

After *abdominal* surgery, a glycerine suppository may be given as early as the second morning, the main result being the passage of flatus which will bring considerable comfort to the patient during the coming day. A mild aperient may be given on the second evening, followed on the fourth day by further suppositories or occasionally an enema if necessary.

After *vaginal* surgery, it is preferable, but not essential, to confine the bowel for three days; straining must be avoided and a gentle bowel action may be assisted by a mild aperient given on the second or third evening, followed the next day by rectal suppositories.

Care of the bladder

Care of the bladder continues to be very important, and must be planned and evaluated as in the first 24 hours after surgery (see page 227).

Urinary output usually reverts to normal within 48 hours of the operation or the removal of an indwelling catheter, although most patients are aware of a bruised feeling at the end of micturition. This is caused by bruising of the bladder and may continue for some six weeks.

An indwelling catheter is removed as instructed by the surgeon; this is usually the seventh day after vaginal surgery, or 48 hours after catheterization in abdominal surgery. It should be removed in the morning to allow bladder function to be assessed before nightfall. There will be three possible outcomes: some patients will pass urine normally; others may appear to do so but have a moderate amount of residual urine; and the third group will have obvious signs of retention (see 'Urinary complications', page 237). Careful observation, accurate recording and interpretation of fluid charts are essential to identify problems.

Should the patient complain of burning at the onset of

micturition, a midstream specimen of urine should be sent to the laboratory. It is not uncommon for the urine to become infected, especially after hysterectomy, and a course of the appropriate antibiotic with a high fluid intake should effect a cure before the patient is discharged.

Care of the abdominal wound

If a drainage tube has been inserted to prevent formation of a haematoma, this is removed as the surgeon instructed, usually after 24 hours.

The dressing may be removed and a plastic spray such as Nobecutane applied, thus enabling the patient to take a bath before the sutures have been removed. Otherwise, the dressing would remain undisturbed until Michel clips or sutures are removed. These are removed from a transverse incision earlier than from a midline incision, but in either case alternate ones are usually left in situ for an extra day. Following their removal, the patient may have a bath and the wound is left dry and exposed to the air.

Care of the vulva

All patients who have had a gynaecological operation need to keep the vulva as clean and fresh as possible, so a vulval and perineal toilet should be carried out three times per day and following defaecation. This is a simple wash of the vulva, groins and perineum with soap and warm water, using a flannel especially reserved for the purpose. A bidet is a welcome aid. The nurse must ensure that the patient has sufficient pads to change often; sterile ones are only really necessary for the first 48 hours after operation.

Specific vulval care will depend on the vaginal discharge present and whether or not there are any perineal sutures.

Vaginal discharge Following ovarian cystectomy or myomectomy there should be no vaginal loss unless the patient has a normal menstrual period. Following hysterectomy or vaginal operations where there is no vaginal pack, vaginal discharge is a small bloodstained loss which gradually decreases until the ninth or tenth day; then as internal sutures dissolve it becomes yellow and increases in amount. This may continue for five to six weeks and will be profuse if there has been much repair work to the vaginal walls. The patient should be warned about this as an unexpected discharge could cause her great anxiety. Should it become bright red, her doctor must be informed immediately.

If there is a vaginal pack, the loss through the pack should be negligible. It normally remains in situ from 24 to 48 hours postoperatively. Following its removal the patient must be observed for the possible onset of bleeding.

Perineal sutures The suture line must be kept as clean and dry as possible. If discomfort is severe, anaesthetic gel applied around the urethral orifice and over the suture line gives relief. Occasionally, there is severe bruising of the perineum and applications of lead lotion or sitting in a bath may be comforting. Because of its rich blood supply the perineum is healed by about the fifth postoperative day, and although the sutures are usually chromic catgut, any which have not dissolved may be removed. This is facilitated by a good light, the patient in the left lateral position and an assistant to raise the buttock. Once the sutures have been removed, a bath twice daily replaces the perineal toilet. Baths may be taken even if there is a catheter in position.

Insertion of soluble pessaries

Vaginal pessaries are sometimes prescribed postoperatively for use either in hospital or once the patient has been sent home, for example nystatin for the treatment of monilial infection, or oestrogen-containing pessaries for post-meno-pausal patients.

Pessaries may be inserted by either the nurse or the patient, but the nurse is responsible to ensure that it is done correctly and she must therefore be certain that the patient understands where and how to insert them.

The patient should empty her bladder. If an applicator is used, she lies in the dorsal position and gently inserts the pessary high up into the posterior fornix of the vagina. Alternatively, she can lie in the left lateral position and the nurse inserts the pessary with her gloved right hand. A vulval pad is applied and the patient remains in bed until the morning. It is helpful to raise the foot of the bed on small blocks.

Rehabilitation

Most gynaecological patients are married women who look forward to returning to the love and security of their own families, but there will be a proportion of single, widowed or divorced women who face adjustment in the less homely atmosphere of a bedsitting room or an old people's home. These patients in particular will experience some feeling of apprehension at the prospect of discharge, and they will probably appreciate the extra care they would receive in a convalescent home.

Surgeons vary in their opinions as to when a patient should be discharged from hospital, but they rarely recommend less than ten days. Where possible, several days' warning of the day of discharge should be given so that the patient can prepare herself mentally as well as physically. Prior to discharge, the house surgeon will carry out a complete abdominal and maybe also a vaginal examination to check that everything is healing satisfactorily.

When the patient leaves she should know that her own doctor will receive a letter from the hospital with information about her treatment, and that she may go to him at any time if she is worried. All her questions about her operation must have been answered, and information given to her such as when to expect her next menstrual period, the length of time that should elapse before she has intercourse and advice about standing, lifting, pushing or pulling heavy weights. Patients who have had vaginal operations should avoid straining and lifting for three months. This may need to be emphasized to women who are independent and tend to fulfil many responsibilities with home, family and work.

The patient needs to understand that the surgeon will wish to see her again in a few weeks or months, and the necessary appointment may be given on discharge or sent through the post.

COMPLICATIONS AFTER GYNAECOLOGICAL SURGERY

Any complication of an anaesthetic or of general surgery is possible after a gynaecological operation. It is all too easy, when familiar with the long and successful operation lists in gynaecology wards, for the nurse to slacken her meticulous standard of care and observation.

The following complications may occur after a gynaecological operation, as in general surgery.

Early complications	*Later complications*
Respiratory failure	Chest infection
Shock	Wound haematoma
Postoperative vomiting	Local infection
Abdominal distention	Burst abdomen
Paralytic ileus	Deep vein thrombosis
	Pulmonary embolus

Complications specific to gynaecology patients are dealt with in more depth.

Haemorrhage Haemorrhage may occur from the abdominal or vaginal vault wound immediately on return from theatre or a few hours later when the blood pressure begins to rise. The warning signs are a rising pulse rate with decreasing volume. In severe haemorrhage the patient quickly becomes pale, restless and sweating, and there is a dramatic fall in blood pressure and pulse volume. The nurse should lose no time in informing the doctor of the first suspicion of haemorrhage.

Vaginal bleeding may be visible before the signs of shock become apparent. For this reason the foot of the bed is only elevated after gynaecological surgery if the condition of the patient specially warrants it, that is, if vomiting occurs when anaesthetized or there is an abnormally low blood pressure.

Pressure may be applied to the bleeding area in the form of a pad and bandage to the abdominal wound, or a pack in the vagina pending the patient's return to the theatre for ligation of blood vessels. Replacement of the fluid loss will be commenced immediately.

Secondary haemorrhage occurs about the eighth or tenth day due to infection. There may be vaginal bleeding and a patient with a small bright red loss should rest in bed for 24 to 48 hours, which should be sufficient to arrest further bleeding. If there is pyrexia and an offensive loss, a vaginal swab should be taken for bacteriological examination and the appropriate antibiotic given. There is usually a slight pyrexia before the haemorrhage, and the temperature chart should be studied carefully at this time. Should a massive haemorrhage occur a vaginal pack would be inserted, the blood loss replaced by transfusion, and the patient returned to theatre for examination and resuturing.

Pelvic haematoma Pelvic haematoma is a more usual complication of a vaginal operation, but following a hysterectomy blood may collect in the fatty tissue between the bladder and pubic bones causing a haematoma. A pyrexia about the seventh to tenth day which falls dramatically with the onset of a purulent vaginal discharge is a characteristic feature. A vaginal swab should be sent for bacteriological examination and an antibiotic given if thought to be necessary. The nurse must see that the vulval area is kept clean and that the vulval pad is changed frequently.

Urinary complications Disturbance of micturition is not uncommon because of the anatomical relationship of the pelvic organs. Any complications usually occur in one of two ways.

Frank retention of urine The patient is unable to pass urine at all and the bladder becomes increasingly distended. The bladder is palpable per abdomen, and may be percussed, but this is unreliable in the obese patient. The patient may or may not have the desire to pass urine, and she will be distressed if she cannot do so. She requires much understanding and patience, which is often difficult to give whilst she incessantly demands to try to use a bedpan, exhausting not only herself but also the nurses. If there is an element of tension, then the running of taps, relief of underlying pain or a mild tranquillizer may have effect. If the bladder is allowed to become overfull, strain is caused on sutures, especially after vaginal repair.

Retention with overflow The patient frequently passes small amounts of urine, but the bladder does not empty and becomes increasingly distended. The nurse must be particularly astute at interpreting the fluid chart to recognize this, because the use of a bedpan may mistakenly be presumed to be a sign of emptying of the bladder. The conventional methods of inducing micturition in the early postoperative period are of little avail in this case, because this is almost entirely a mechanical problem to which only time provides the answer.

Treatment of both types of retention is catheterization. The differential diagnosis of retention with overflow is made when the residual urine immediately after passing urine is more than 100 ml. Some surgeons prefer repeated catheterization, but most recommend that the bladder be drained continuously for at least 48 hours to allow it to rest. A second attempt to establish the act of normal micturition is usually successful. The patient may be asked to pass urine and be catheterized immediately afterwards, in order to measure the residual urine, and if this is between 100 ml and 300 ml she should be recatheterized and the procedure repeated each 24 hours until the amount is reduced to normal (less than 100 ml).

A urinary antiseptic such as nitrofurantoin 50–100 mg four times a day may be ordered as a prophylactic measure. Retention of urine is not unexpected, especially after vaginal operations, and it is important for all to realize this so that a 'major crisis' does not develop if normal micturition is not established immediately.

On the rare occasion that the bladder is injured, blood-stained urine may be passed; it is important for the nurse to be certain that this is haematuria and not contamination from the vaginal loss. A large swab should be used to occlude the vaginal orifice whilst urine is passed, care being taken to remove it afterwards.

Even more rarely, the ureter may be ligatured or injured, this is possible during a Wertheim's hysterectomy. It is suspected if there is pain in the loin and abdomen, associated with a reduced urinary output. If the condition is bilateral, the patient's condition rapidly deteriorates.

Later urinary complications

Infection When the patient has no indwelling catheter, urinary infections such as cystitis and pyelonephritis sometimes occur. These may be due to bruising of the bladder at operation, predisposing to difficulties of micturition and subsequent infection.

When the patient has a catheter, urinary infection may occur despite meticulous catheterization and the use of urinary antiseptics. Management would be to ensure free drainage, increase fluid intake, culture the organism and give the appropriate antibiotic.

Other urinary complications are unlikely to persist longer than the first 24 hours after abdominal surgery, but following vaginal surgery further problems may be encountered.

Retention If retention of urine persists for some weeks, as occasionally happens after vaginal surgery, the pressure of the catheter may cause oedema of the urethral epithelium or a urethral stricture. A variety of treatments may be adopted: some surgeons favour the use of carbachol by injection as this causes constriction of the bladder muscle and the voiding of urine; others attempt to re-educate the bladder by spigoting the catheter and releasing it at gradually increasing intervals. In the case of a urethral stricture, dilatation of the urethra under a general anaesthetic usually relieves this.

Incontinence Apparent incontinence once the catheter has been removed should be reported immediately as it may indicate a vesicovaginal fistula (page 271). It could also be due to retention with overflow, but if careful observations have been made, retention would have been noted before reaching this stage.

Certain other complications may not be discovered until the patient visits the outpatient department some three months after operation.

Dyspareunia This can be caused by low-grade infection, scarring, or a vaginal stricture.

Recurrent stress incontinence A relapse occurs in 5% of cases.

Vaginal fistulae Vesicovaginal, rectovaginal or urethro-vaginal fistulae may occur, especially where there is carcinoma (see Chapter 24).

Vaginal vault prolapse Vaginal vault prolapse is a late complication of abdominal hysterectomy and a rare one, but it can be caused by an enterocele (see Chapter 26).

FURTHER READING

FISH, E.J. (1979) *Surgical Nursing*, 10th ed., Chapters 2, 8, and 15. London: Baillière Tindall.

20 Gynaecological Examination

Gynaecological examination has three parts:
1. *taking the history*, to identify the problem
2. *physical examination*, to assess the condition
3. *discussion*, to plan and evaluate care.

Nurses and doctors working in gynaecological departments become so accustomed to the extent to which a patient is exposed during examination, that they tend not to notice this. Patients always notice. From the moment the patient walks into the gynaecology department she feels vulnerable.

The role of the nurse is to reassure, by her words and her actions, which should enable the patient to cooperate with all three parts of the examination. For example, it is the nurse's responsibility not only to close doors or curtains, but also to assure the patient that they will remain closed, so that her privacy will be preserved. By showing understanding, the nurse can gain the confidence and cooperation of the patient. This in turn will ensure that better care is given, because:

1. the problem is identified more easily when the patient is relaxed enough to give a coherent history
2. the condition is assessed more accurately when the patient allows thorough physical examination
3. the patient is happier with her care when she is enabled to participate in discussion to plan and evaluate it.

Taking the history

All details of history taken at an antenatal clinic (see Chapter

4) are important in a gynaecological examination. Particular attention is paid to the following.

Menstrual history because this is an important sign of gynaecological problems.

Obstetric history, especially trauma or infection which can often cause gynaecological conditions.

Urinary problems because of the interrelation of organs in such close proximity.

Endocrine disorders because these may interfere with hormone profiles.

Physical examination

This is carried out in a warm, private room which is free from draughts. The light must be good, so an adjustable lamp or torch is most convenient.

Throughout the examination, the nurse's duty is twofold.

1. *To help the patient.* This means explaining what is to be done *before* the examination, thereby gaining her cooperation *during* it. The nurse should imagine how the patient feels and allay each anxiety with explanations, whilst also preventing unnecessary embarrassment by preventing undue exposure whenever the doctor forgets. If the patient is frightened and holds herself tense, the gynaecologist will be hampered and examination may be painful. Gentle breathing with the mouth open will help her to relax her muscles, so making the examination easier.

2. *To assist the doctor.* This means preparing the patient and the trolley (see 'Special Requirements', page 247).

The patient should empty her bladder. Clothing should be removed and her gown or nightdress should be loosely fitting to allow full examination by the doctor. The doctor should be told if she is menstruating, and any pad removed saved for inspection.

The nurse must be able to place the patient promptly in any of the special positions described later, ensuring comfort to the patient and convenience for the doctor.

A light sheet should be used and folded appropriately to expose no more of the patient than is necessary for vaginal examination. If the breasts were previously examined, they should *always* be covered before exposing the lower half of the patient.

When the doctor has finished, the nurse must ensure that the vulva is dry and that the patient is comfortable, before clearing away and labelling the various specimens.

Discussion

This should preferably be done after the patient has dressed and made herself feel human again. Dressing actually gives her valuable time on her own to gather her thoughts together and recall any questions to ask the doctor. Her greatest embarrassment is now over, so this no longer dominates her mind, and she feels more able to think clearly.

Any investigations are arranged and possible treatment is explained clearly. When appropriate, explanation is also given about the effect of the patient's condition on other aspects of her life, such as sexual relationships, fertility, or mood changes.

POSITIONS USED FOR GYNAECOLOGICAL EXAMINATIONS

Dorsal position (Fig. 20.1)

This is used for abdominal, vulval, vaginal and bimanual examinations of the pelvis.

The patient lies on her back with the head supported on one pillow. The knees are flexed and apart (abducted).

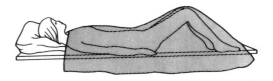

Fig. 20.1 Dorsal position.

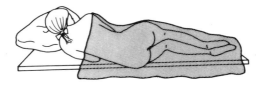

Fig. 20.2 Left lateral position.

Left lateral position (Fig. 20.2)

This may be used for vulval, vaginal and rectal examinations, for taking swabs of the vagina, or for delivery.

The patient lies on her left side with the buttocks well to the edge of the bed, and one pillow under her head.

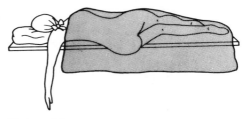

Fig. 20.3 Sim's position.

Sim's position (Fig. 20.3)

This may be convenient for examination of the vagina, insertion of a pessary or pack, and other vaginal treatments, as it gives rather easier access.

This is an exaggerated left lateral position. The left arm is placed behind the back, the right arm is flexed towards the head and the right knee is flexed. One pillow is placed on the far side of the bed for the head. Thus the patient is in a semiprone position with the pelvis and trunk tilted towards the bed.

Great care must be taken in arranging the left arm, as it can cause pain in the shoulder.

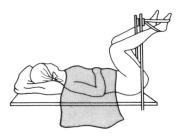

Fig. 20.4 Lithotomy position.

Lithotomy position (Fig. 20.4)
This is used for operations on the vagina, vulva or rectum, and for forceps delivery.

The patient lies on her back and the legs are fully abducted with her heels supported in stirrups specially adjusted on the side of the bed or operating table.

Special points
1. Socks should be worn to protect the ankles.
2. Both legs must be flexed simultaneously on to the abdomen and then the feet moved to the outer side of the poles. If each leg is moved separately, sacroiliac strain is caused.
3. If the legs are not fully abducted, pressure from the leg rests may obstruct the venous return.

Once the patient is positioned, the bottom part of the table is lowered and the patient's buttocks are lifted to the edge. For operative procedures, drapes are used to provide a sterile field.

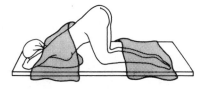

Fig. 20.5 Genupectoral position.

Genupectoral position (knee–chest) (Fig. 20.5)
This is used for culdoscopy, and in obstetrics to relieve the pressure following prolapse of the umbilical cord.

The patient kneels on the bed, bends forward and rests her head and shoulders on a pillow so that her thighs are in a vertical position, and the pelvis is as high as possible. This displaces the contents of the pelvis towards the diaphragm and relieves the pressure.

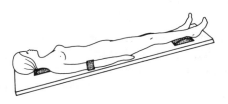

Fig. 20.6 Trendelenburg position.

Trendelenburg position (Fig. 20.6)

This is used for pelvic operations such as hysterectomy, oophorectomy and caesarean section.

The anaesthetized patient lies recumbent on the theatre table, which is then tilted head downwards. This allows the abdominal contents to fall against the diaphragm and gives better access to the pelvic cavity.

SPECIAL REQUIREMENTS FOR GYNAECOLOGICAL EXAMINATION

Routine vaginal examination

Paper towel for under the buttocks
Disposable gloves
Bowl of lotion
Lubricant, e.g. Hibitane cream
Specula—Sims', Cusco's and Ferguson's (See Figs. 20.7, 20.8 and 20.10)
Bowl of warm water for warming the specula
Wool swabs and swab-holding forceps
Receptacle for used instruments
Disposable bag for used gloves and swabs

Aseptic technique is not normally used for vaginal examination unless the patient is aborting, in labour, or postpartum. In this case, all the above apparatus must be sterile and, in addition, vulsellum forceps (see Fig. 20.12) may be required.

Additional requirements for obtaining vaginal or cervical specimens

Sterile swab stick
Stuart's medium
Ayre spatula (Fig. 20.9)
Microscope slides and cover slips
Pathological request forms

A high vaginal swab is taken to isolate organisms in cases of suspected genital tract infection.

The patient should be placed in the left lateral or Sim's position and the light arranged so that it will shine into the vagina when the speculum is inserted. A towel is placed under the buttocks and, after the nurse has washed her hands, the vulva is swabbed and dried. The speculum is lubricated and inserted gently in a backward direction, the labia being separated with the left hand and the speculum held in the right hand. When the cervix can be seen, the swab is inserted through the speculum and the vaginal vault swabbed. The swab is returned to its container, the speculum removed, the vulva dried and the patient left comfortable. The specimen is labelled and dispatched to the laboratory without delay.

Additional requirements for obtaining Papanicolaou's smear

Ayre spatulae (Fig. 20.9)
Microscope slides
Diamond pencil
Container with fixation fluid for slide
Histological request forms

All cervices shed their most superficial layer of squamous cells into the vagina and new cells are produced from the

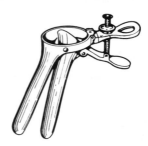

Fig. 20.7 Cusco's speculum.

deeper layers. It is possible by means of an Ayre spatula to pick up these cells in secretions taken from the cervix. The secretion is smeared on a glass slide and immediately immersed in a solution of alcohol and ether. This is sent to the laboratory for microscopic examination for abnormal (malignant) cells.

INSTRUMENTS USED FOR GYNAECOLOGICAL EXAMINATION

Cusco's speculum (Fig. 20.7) is used to expose the cervix for inspection or to take samples such as cervical secretions. The speculum is lubricated and inserted in the closed position into the vagina, rotated and then opened to separate the anterior and posterior vaginal walls. The patient is in the dorsal position.

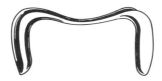

Fig. 20.8 Sim's speculum.

Sim's speculum (Fig. 20.8) is used to retract the posterior vaginal wall and expose the cervix, for example when packing or painting the vagina. The end should be lubricated and passed along the posterior vaginal wall. The patient is in the left lateral position

Ayre spatula (Fig. 20.9) is used to take a Papanicolaou's smear; the reverse end may be used to obtain a specimen from the vaginal fornices. It is a wooden or plastic spatula, so designed that the longer portion (A) is passed into the cervical canal and rotated. This collects cells from the

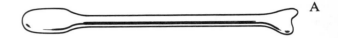

A

Fig. 20.9 Ayre spatula.

squamocolumnar junction, the point where carcinoma is most likely to commence.

Ferguson's speculum (Fig. 20.10) is used when more support is required than can be given by the bivalve speculum. It is essentially just a metal tube which supports prolapsed vaginal walls to allow a view of the cervix. The patient is in the left lateral position.

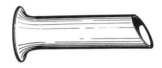

Fig. 20.10 Ferguson's speculum.

Auvard's speculum (Fig. 20.11) is a weighted vaginal retractor and is only used in the operating theatre when the patient is anaesthetized.

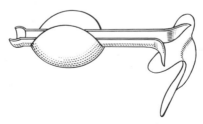

Fig. 20.11 Auvard's speculum.

Vulsellum forceps (Fig. 20.12) have large teeth which can grasp the cervix and allow traction to be exerted durin;

procedures requiring the passage of an instrument through
the cervical canal.

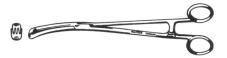

Fig. 20.12 Vulsellum forceps.

Hegar's dilators (Fig. 20.13) may be single or double
ended and consist of a set of progressive sizes (1 to 16). They
are passed through the cervical canal in turn in order to dilate
it.

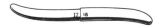

Fig. 20.13 Hegar's dilator.

Uterine curettes (Figs 20.14 and 20.15) may have a sharp
or blunt end, may be double ended or flushing. These are
passed into the uterus in order to scrape a specimen from the
lining. The flushing curette allows for irrigation at the same
time.

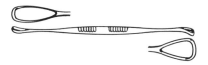

Fig. 20.14 Uterine curette.

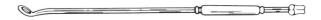

Fig. 20.15 Flushing curette.

Ovum forceps (Fig. 20.16) are shaped like two spoons, which grasp the ovum or other debris and aid its removal from the uterine cavity.

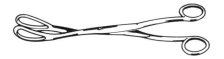

Fig. 20.16 Ovum forceps.

Uterine sound (Fig. 20.17) is a long, thin instrument with graduations. This is passed into the uterus in order to measure its length.

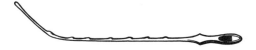

Fig. 20.17 Uterine sound.

Female bladder sound (Fig. 20.18) has no graduations and is fatter and shorter than a male bladder sound. It is used to estimate the size of the bladder.

Fig. 20.18 Female bladder sound.

21 Disorders of the Vulva

Disorders of the vulva are very distressing to a patient. She cannot be helped by sharing her troubles, because she is too embarrassed to mention them: she is often too afraid even to seek help from the doctor. Vulval itching may drive her to distraction, but our society does not allow polite ladies to touch. Unlike more sociable disorders, such as a broken leg, vulval disorders are fraught with embarrassment.

The nurse is the one person who can show understanding, because patients know that nurses have seen these sorts of problems before and are therefore much less inhibited in talking about them. A nurse is thus able to help by bringing practical comfort as well as by giving informed words of reassurance.

THE VULVA

The vulva is composed of the following structures (Fig. 21.1).

The mons veneris The mons veneris is a pad of fat lying in front of the symphysis pubis, covered by skin and, after puberty, short hair.

The labia majora The labia majora are two rounded folds of fatty tissue and skin which pass downwards and backwards from the mons veneris to merge into the perineum.

The labia minora The labia minora are two smaller folds

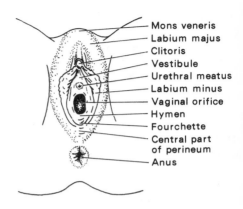

Fig. 21.1 The external genital organs.

within the labia majora which encircle the vestibule and ar joined posteriorly by a thin fold of skin, the fourchette.

The vestibule The vestibule is the narrow cleft between th labia minora containing the vaginal and urethral orifices.

The clitoris The clitoris is a sensitive area of highly vascula erectile tissue extending inwards for about 2 cm.

The urethral meatus The urethral meatus is a small vertica slit, sometimes difficult to identify, lying 2 cm below th clitoris. There is a dimple on either side which helps i locating the orifice.

The vaginal orifice The vaginal orifice, or introitus vaginae occupies the lower two-thirds of the vestibule. In the virgi this is closed by the hymen.

The hymen The hymen is a perforated membrane over th

vaginal orifice, its function being to prevent the entry of urine into the vagina.

Bartholin's glands The two Bartholin's glands lie on either side of the posterior part of the vaginal orifice. They are compound racemose glands whose ducts pass inwards to open on to the surface just medial to the labia minora. They secrete mucus which lubricates and moistens the external genitalia.

Between the vulva and the anus is the area of skin called the perineum.

INFLAMMATION

Vulval irritation and inflammation

As with skin anywhere else in the body, the vulva is subjected to inflammatory conditions such as eczema, psoriasis and allergic conditions precipitated by soap or underwear.

Systemic diseases, including diabetes mellitus, urticaria, some of the reticuloses and any condition resulting in jaundice, will cause a generalized irritation (pruritus).

Local conditions arising from poor hygiene, vaginal discharge, pediculosis pubis and threadworms will cause irritation and scratching and are prone to secondary infection.

Acute vulvitis is not common, but may be caused by bacteria or fungi. The most common form is secondary to a vaginal discharge. This tends to cause soreness as well as irritation, oedema and erythema.

Treatment consists of frequent baths or cleansing of the vulva area, drying carefully and dusting liberally with a fine, unscented talcum powder. The patient should be encouraged to wear loose cotton underclothing.

Furunculosis

Small staphylococcal abscesses may occur at the base of the

hair follicles in the pubic or vulval area. These are painful and difficult to control. Careful washing with hexachlorophene soap may be helpful, or exposure to ultraviolet light. Since they tend to recur, systemic treatment with an antibiotic may be necessary.

Intertrigo

Intertrigo, or chafing, occurs where two skin surfaces rub together. The skin macerates, becomes inflamed, hot and glazed in appearance. The surface may be rubbed off and the underlying tissue become infected. The patient may complain of pruritus and a burning sensation. She should be advised to wash and dry the vulva carefully, and either to dust with talcum powder or apply thick calamine lotion liberally. Soft loose underwear will help to avoid friction and assist in healing. If the problem is exacerbated by obesity, the patient may be advised to lose some weight.

Varicose veins

Varicose veins of the vulva are rarely seen except as a complication of pregnancy (see Chapter 5).

Urethral caruncle

A caruncle is a small, bright red swelling on the posterior lip of the urinary meatus which bleeds very easily and may be confused with vaginal bleeding (Fig. 21.2). The symptoms are pain, frequency of micturition, bleeding and dyspareunia. The treatment is cauterization or excision of the lesion, but the caruncle is likely to recur. Oestrogen may be prescribed when the condition is associated with post-menopausal vaginitis.

Bartholin's cyst or abscess

A cyst may form if the duct of a Bartholin's gland becomes blocked, for example by infection or injury during childbirth

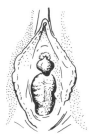

Fig. 21.2 Urethral caruncle.

The cyst can rapidly become infected and the fluid turn to pus, forming a Bartholin's abscess (Fig. 21.3). This is a very painful swelling beneath the posterior fold of the labium majorum.

Treatment involves surgical excision or marsupialization (making into a small pouch that opens on to the skin). Systemic treatment with antibiotics may also be necessary, so if there is any discharge a swab should be taken for culture. Postoperatively, hot baths should be given twice daily. The area should be dried with a sterile piece of gauze both after bathing and after micturition.

The patient is usually discharged within 48 hours.

WHITE LESIONS OF THE VULVA

Kraurosis vulvae

Kraurosis vulvae is a degenerative condition occurring in elderly women. There is progressive atrophy of the vulva, with loss of hair and the skin is then smooth and parchment-like in appearance. It produces severe irritation which may be relieved by coal-tar ointments, zinc and castor-oil cream or hydrocortisone ointment. Systemic treatment with stil-boestrol may be effective. This is not a cancerous condition.

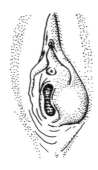

Fig. 21.3 Bartholin's abscess.

Leukoplakia vulvae

Leukoplakia vulvae is a premalignant condition affecting the skin of the vulva and adjacent areas. It almost always occurs after the menopause, and at least 50% of cases eventually progress to a squamous cell carcinoma.

The clinical picture is difficult to distinguish from kraurosis, as the only symptom as a rule is severe irritation of the vulva. As the condition develops the vulval skin shows wrinkled, scaly white patches which are raised and dry. Later, cracks appear which may become infected: it is in these cracks that malignant change can occur.

Treatment is first a biopsy to eliminate malignant changes, then an effort is made to relieve the irritation and allow the fissures to heal. If this fails, simple vulvectomy will be necessary (page 260), and the patient is usually very grateful for the relief this brings.

NEW GROWTH

Papilloma

These warty growths may be simple or multiple, they are

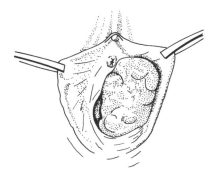

Fig. 21.4 Carcinoma of the vulva.

benign and non-venereal although sometimes misnamed venereal warts. They generally occur in association with leucorrhoea, pregnancy or poor hygiene. The usual location is the posterior part of the vulva, perineum and buttocks and occasionally they are found in the vagina. Treatment is to improve the standard of hygiene, eliminate leucorrhoea if present and apply podophylin in alcohol. Those occurring in pregnancy usually disappear spontaneously within hours of delivery.

Carcinoma

Carcinoma of the vulva generally occurs in women over 50 years of age (Fig. 21.4). It is usually a primary growth, and in most instances preceded by leukoplakia. The patient becomes aware of intense irritation of the vulva which bleeds on any friction or scratching, and she may also notice a small pimple-like growth which increases in size. The condition is not usually painful unless secondary infection occurs.

On examination, shallow ulceration or a firm lump may be found, the diagnosis can be confirmed if necessary by a biopsy. Treatment is by radical vulvectomy (page 261), but the prognosis over five years is not good.

OPERATIONS ON THE VULVA

Simple or local vulvectomy

Vulvectomy varies in extent from simple excision of the labia for intractable pruritus vulvae to an excision of the mons veneris, clitoris and labia for leukoplakia. One incision is made around the whole vulva, and another around the vaginal introitus including the urethral meatus above. All tissue between these incisions is removed and the skin edges sutured (Fig. 21.5).

Preoperative care is given as detailed in Chapter 19. When assessing the patient's needs, special consideration must be given to her need for reassurance by explanations of the exact nature of the operation. The nurse may find that a diagram is helpful to show which parts will be removed, or she could, when shaving the vulva, point to the areas.

The vulva is the outer sign to a person that she is female— at the moment she was born, the vulva meant 'It's a girl!' When that is removed a woman has special needs for caring information: married women especially must be reassured that the vagina will remain. Sexual intercourse after simple vulvectomy is possible, usually after at least three months but depending on the amount of postoperative stenosis. Each

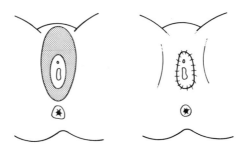

Fig. 21.5 Area of tissue removed in simple vulvectomy.

patient should be told *pre*operatively that she will be advised about this at her follow-up appointment.

Postoperatively, a catheter may be in place for a few days, to help to keep the wound clean and dry. Black silk sutures are removed on the seventh day.

Radical vulvectomy

A radical vulvectomy is an extensive operation performed for carcinoma of the vulva. The vulva, clitoris, mons veneris and perineal tissue are excised, combined with a block dissection of the superficial and deep inguinal and femoral glands (Fig. 21.6). If the skin edges cannot be approximated, as is often the case, they are left to granulate.

Preoperative care is given as for simple vulvectomy, with appropriate amendments in explanations. It is important to prepare the patient for a lengthy stay in hospital.

Postoperative care is based on the principles of maintaining the patient's morale through a long and difficult period of recovery; and keeping the wound clean, dry and free from tension. Healing by primary intention is rarely possible because of the scanty amount of skin available. Sometimes the area will be left to heal by granulation and covered with tulle gras. If the skin edges have been closed, breakdown is very likely. A Readivac type of drainage tube on each side

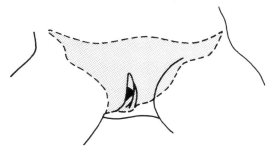

Fig. 21.6 Area of tissue removed in radical vulvectomy.

262 Obstetrics and Gynaecology

may help to relieve tension. The dressings, apart from the tulle gras, will require changing frequently. Radiant heat, Eusol dressings and penicillin powder may be used to assist granulation where necessary. A large bed cradle will relieve the pressure of the bedclothes, and when moving the patient she should be turned with her knees together to prevent strain on the suture line. Passive physiotherapy must be started as soon as possible as complications are likely to occur following a long anaesthetic. A self-retaining catheter will be in position for five to seven days, and analgesics will be given at regular intervals. The patient is allowed up on the second day, but because of the analgesics feels surprisingly little pain. Trust and confidence in the nursing and medical staff are of paramount importance as the extent of the incision, appearance of the wound and disfigurement of the vulval region can be a tremendous shock to the patient, however carefully she was prepared beforehand. The nursing care calls for tremendous teamwork and it is this that makes the gradual progress towards recovery so rewarding for all concerned.

22 Disorders of the Vagina

Disorders of the vagina have a strong psychological and emotional effect because the implications of the disorder reach far beyond the physiological state. The vagina is important to the patient for a variety of reasons. First, it is an area of privacy and intimacy in terms of her sexual life. Secondly, its well-being is vital to her fertility, both to receive spermatozoa and eventually to act as the birth canal during parturition. To some people in our culture it is considered as something 'dirty' because it is the passage for secretions and debris during menstruation and postpartum.

The nurse must consider the patient's needs in relation to all of these aspects because disorders of the vagina are more threatening to the patient herself than a physiological condition, however simple it may seem to the nurse.

THE VAGINA

The vagina is a fibromuscular canal, sloping upwards and backwards from the introitus to the uterus. The posterior wall measures about 10 cm in length, being 2.5 cm longer than the anterior wall because of the protrusion of the cervix anteriorly. The cervix divides the vaginal vault into four arches, or fornices, named, according to their positions, anterior, posterior, and two lateral fornices.

The vaginal walls are normally in apposition, but are easily separated. They are composed of four layers.

1. A lining of squamous epithelium (modified skin), pink in

colour and thrown into transverse folds, or rugae, which allow great distension without tearing.

2. Elastic connective tissue which is highly vascular.

3. A muscle layer with the inner fibres arranged circularly and the outer ones longitudinally.

4. An outer encircling layer of connective tissue which contains blood vessels, nerves and lymphatics. The blood supply is from several branches of the internal iliac arteries.

Adjacent to the vagina are the following organs.

Bladder base—related to the anterior fornix.

Ureters and uterine vessels—related to the lateral fornices.

Peritoneum and pouch of Douglas—related to the posterior fornix.

Urethra—related to the anterior wall.

Rectum and, lower down, perineal body—related to the posterior wall.

Normal vaginal discharges

The vagina contains no glands but is lubricated by fluid from two sources: the cervical glands which secrete mucus, and a serous transudation from the blood vessels.

The normal vaginal secretions do not cause irritation and the amount is insufficient to require a pad. The character of the discharges changes according to the days of the menstrual cycle:

approx. number of days:

1–4	menstruation
5–11	thin, white secretion
12–14	ovulatory mucus: clear, similar to egg white
15–28	white and mucoid, increasing in amount

During the reproductive years, certain commensals, the lactobacilli, ferment glycogen stored in the epithelium and produce an acid medium (pH 4.5) in which many bacteria cannot flourish. These lactobacilli are only present under the influence of oestrogen, therefore before puberty and after the menopause when oestrogen levels are low, the vagina is less acid (pH 7). Thus, the vagina acts as an effective barrier against ascending infection during the childbearing years.

Abnormal vaginal discharges

A patient may go to the doctor because she becomes aware of abnormal vaginal discharge; that is, if she notices that the amount has increased, or that there is an offensive smell, or that it causes vulval irritation. Vaginal discharge is not a disease in itself, but a sign of other abnormality. The possible causes are:

1. vaginitis, including that caused by foreign bodies (page 267)
2. cervicitis (Chapter 24)
3. pelvic inflammatory disease (Chapter 27)
4. carcinoma of the cervix or body or the uterus (Chapter 24)
5. Vaginal fistulae (pp. 270–271)
6. Venereal disease (Chapter 23)

Patients who complain of vaginal discharge must be examined thoroughly to ensure that the treatment is appropriate to the cause. Management of these patients is therefore discussed with each causative condition.

CONGENITAL ABNORMALITIES

The vagina may be involved with the uterus in certain abnormalities (page 306) resulting in a double vagina. There may be absence or atresia of the vagina and the hymen may be imperforate. Some abnormalities may be corrected by surgery. Congenital absence of part or all of the vagina may be associated with absence of the uterus or with rudimentary organs. The condition is often discovered around the age of 17, when investigations into amenorrhoea are being made. This may have serious repercussions if the woman is contemplating marriage, and surgery may be undertaken to construct an artificial vagina (page 273). This is a long and difficult task, and aims to provide as normal a physical side as possible to married life.

Cryptomenorrhoea

Cryptomenorrhoea means 'concealed menstruation'; that is, menstruation occurs but the blood loss is trapped in the vagina behind an obstruction—usually an imperforate hymen or vaginal atresia.

The patient consults a gynaecologist if she is concerned at the (apparent) failure of the onset of menstruation; or she may have an episode of acute retention of urine if the mass of blood in the vagina (haematocolpos) presses on the bladder neck. There may be a history of regular monthly pain. On examination, the hymen is seen to be tense, blue and bulging. On rectal examination a mass can be felt anteriorly (Fig. 22.1). The condition is usually diagnosed before the collection of altered blood distends the uterus (haematometra) and the uterine tubes (haematosalpinx).

Treatment Hymenectomy is a simple incision of the hymen, which allows the stale blood to drain away; if there is atresia of the vagina, more extensive surgery may be necessary. However small the operation, the nurse must remember that these patients are young girls who are experiencing a whole spectrum of emotions, not only at their first proper period but also at its traumatic onset.

Postoperatively, attention to vulval toilet, sterile pads and general hygiene is very important, since stale blood is an ideal breeding ground for bacteria, and infection can readily occur. This is actually an excellent opportunity to teach the

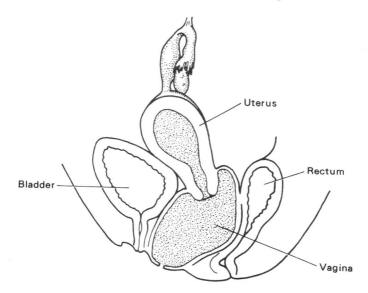

Fig. 22.1 Cryptomenorrhoea.

patient about the importance of good hygiene during normal menstruation.

INFLAMMATION

Vaginitis or inflammation of the vagina may occur at any age.

Vaginitis before puberty

The commonest condition before puberty is vulvovaginitis. Soiled, tight clothing and threadworms may cause irritation and predispose to scratching. The skin of the vulva and vagina is easily damaged by young girls scratching themselves or putting foreign bodies such as beads into the vagina. Infection may follow due to bacteria, monilia, or occasionally from the gonococcus (see Chapter 23).

Vaginitis during reproductive life

In the adult woman only two forms of vaginitis are seen, both caused by organisms which flourish in an acid medium. However, the possibility of gonorrhoea must always be considered because although the organism does not invade the vagina itself, there is a copious discharge from urethritis or cervicitis (see Chapter 23).

Trichomonas vaginalis This condition causes the patient a great deal of distress. She complains of vulval irritation, vaginal discharge, dyspareunia, and sometimes urinary frequency and dysuria. On examination, the vaginal introitus and vaginal walls are very inflamed. There is a profuse greenish-yellow discharge which is offensive and often frothy. There are small punctate haemorrhagic areas on the cervix and adjacent tissues. For confirmation of the diagnosis, a sample of the discharge is taken either with a swab for culture or with a platinum loop for immediate microscopic examination.

The usual treatment is metronidazole (Flagyl) 200 mg daily, by mouth for ten days. The patient should be advised to wash the vulva frequently and to wear clean underclothing each day. If it is necessary for a pad to be worn, it should be changed at least three times a day, or even more often. Intercourse should be avoided until treatment is successfully completed. *Trichomonas vaginalis* is commonly, but not exclusively, transmitted by sexual intercourse and unless both partners are treated it is liable to recur. It is a cause of non-specific urethritis in the male.

In a few instances when treatment with metronidazole fails, arsenical compounds may be ordered. Acetarsol (Stovarsol, SVC) pessaries are inserted high in the vagina over a period of two to six weeks.

Monilial infection *Candida albicans* is a yeast-like fungus, commonly present in the upper respiratory, alimentary and female genital tracts; occasionally, it becomes pathogenic and it can produce a wide variety of disorders including thrush, vulvovaginitis and dermatitis.

Infection occurs more readily when the vagina is less acid; that is, when there is interference with the normal action of the commensal lactobacilli on glycogen (page 265). Examples are:

1. diabetes mellitus, when glycogen levels are higher
2. pregnancy, because mild glycosuria is common
3. prolonged treatment with broad spectrum antibiotics, because this radically alters commensals in the vagina.

The patient complains of pruritus, burning sensation, urinary frequency, dysuria and sometimes dyspareunia. On examination, the vulva is red and swollen, and a whitish curd-like exudate adheres to the inner surface of the labia. The vagina is pale and dry and in the rugal folds is a tenacious exudate the consistency of cream cheese.

There are a number of local treatments which are effective, such as nystatin (Nystan), amphotericin B (Fungilin), noxy-thiolin (Gynaflex) and clotrimazole (Canesten). The patient must be taught how to insert the pessaries high into the vagina at night. This can be done either using an applicator, or with a gloved hand, as one would insert a rectal suppository. A vulval pad should be applied because the pessary usually dissolves and escapes from the vagina after a few hours. Once more the patient should be given advice regarding vulval cleanliness and underclothing. Painting the vagina with gentian violet 1% aqueous solution is very effective but this will stain the patient's clothing permanently.

Vaginitis after the menopause

Senile vaginitis may occur in elderly women because with low oestrogen levels the vaginal acidity is lowered in the absence of lactobacilli. The vaginal endothelium thins, shallow ulcerations may occur, sometimes accompanied by bleeding, followed in some cases by a secondary bacterial infection. The patient may complain of soreness and dyspareunia.

Oestrogen is usually given to encourage the growth of normal commensals. Oestrogen-containing vaginal cream or pessaries may be applied locally, or alternatively oestrogens may be given by mouth.

Any patient with vaginal bleeding after the menopause should be investigated for the possibility of malignant disease.

TRAUMA

Vaginal fistulae

Fistulae occur between the urinary tract and the vagina and between the vagina and rectum (Fig. 22.2). In the United Kingdom they result from malignant disease and its treatment, or from operations in the pelvis for other causes. In countries where obstetric help is inadequate they all too frequently occur as a result of obstructed labour and continued pressure

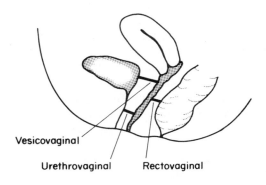

Vesicovaginal

Urethrovaginal   Rectovaginal

Fig. 22.2 Vaginal fistulae.

of the fetal head against the symphysis pubis and sacrum.

Carcinoma of the cervix may invade the bladder or rectum causing fistulae, necrosis may follow irradiation for such a growth. Damage may occur even in the most skilled hands during a Wertheim's hysterectomy.

The symptoms of a fistula are incontinence unrelated to posture, stress or any other factor. The patient is miserable and uncomfortable as her underwear is never dry, the vulva becomes sore and excoriated, an unpleasant odour develops however meticulous the hygienic care may be.

Vesicovaginal fistula

Vesicovaginal fistula may close spontaneously if a self-retaining catheter is passed and continuous drainage adopted for two weeks. If this is not successful, it is advisable to wait until the oedema and fibrosis are reduced. The fistula is repaired vaginally.

Ureterovaginal fistula

In the case of ureterovaginal fistula it would probably be necessary to reimplant the ureter into the bladder. This is an abdominal operation.

Rectovaginal fistula

Rectovaginal fistula would be repaired as a vaginal operation after oedema and fibrosis have resolved.

Following malignant disease, treatment can only be palliative, and may mean transplantation of the ureters or a colostomy.

NEW GROWTH

New growths are rare, and malignant conditions are usually associated with spread from a cervical or pelvic carcinoma. The treatment is determined by the site of the primary lesion.

OPERATIONS ON THE VAGINA

Enlargement of the vaginal orifice

Enlargement of the vaginal orifice is indicated when the small introitus causes dyspareunia or even apareunia.

When severe dyspareunia is of physiological origin, naturally, psychological strain and frustration are likely to accompany it. When psychological factors cause the problem, physiological change may appear to occur—for example, a woman can be so tense that she can prevent the vaginal muscles from stretching. It is thus very important to assess whether an apparently small introitus is caused by physiological or psychological factors.

Operations which may be performed are as follows.

Hymenectomy—excision of the hymen (see page 266).

Dilatation of vaginal orifice—by digital means or vaginal dilators.

Fenton's operation—the principle is to divide all the fibres of the perineal body except the anal sphincter. A longitudinal incision is made through the skin and muscle of the perineal body, and the longitudinal wound is then closed transversely (Fig. 22.3).

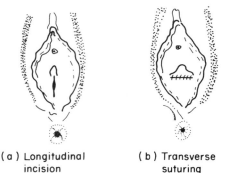

   (a) Longitudinal   (b) Transverse
        incision   suturing

Fig. 22.3 Fenton's operation.

Following these operations, patients may return to the ward with a vaginal dilator in position, kept in place by a T-bandage. It may be appropriate to wait until the patient is sufficiently awake to see the size of the dilator when it is removed, if there is an underlying psychological factor, in which case it would be therapeutic to actually let her see the size to which her vagina has been enlarged.

Intercourse should be avoided for about six weeks, by which time the area is well healed.

Vaginoplasty

Vaginoplasty is the construction of an artificial vagina, and is indicated when a patient is prevented from coitus by congenital absence of the vagina or by contractures due to injury. Operations which may be performed are as follows.

McIndoe–Bannister operation is carried out with the assistance of a plastic surgeon. A plastic mould is covered with skin from the thigh, forming a pouch. This is inserted into an incision between the urethra and rectum, and is kept in place by suturing the labia minora. The mould must be kept in situ for several months, and one it is removed the patient should be given a vaginal dilator. In order to prevent contraction of the new vagina, she should be shown how to pass this daily whenever she does not have intercourse.

Williams' operation is the formation of a cul-de-sac by splitting the labia majora down to the perineal muscles. The resultant U-shape is resutured longitudinally, in two layers such that the anterior wall of the new 'vagina' is the vulva, and the posterior wall is the restructured labia.

FURTHER READING

PARKER, M.J. & STUCKE, V.S. (1982) *Microbiology for Nurses*, 6th ed., London: Baillière Tindall.

23 Venereal Diseases

Venereal diseases are diseases which are spread by sexual intercourse. Since the Venereal Disease Act in 1917 all patients suffering from such diseases have been treated under medical supervision in a special clinic where the treatment is confidential and free of charge; the service antedated the National Health Service by some 30 years. Of the women attending, 80% suffer from some non-venereal condition and only the remainder from a true venereal disease.

Venereal diseases are not notifiable in England as it is considered that patients are more likely to go voluntarily for their treatment if the clinics are run in conjunction with general hospitals. It is of great importance that clinics are open at times suitable for the patient who has to work during the day. Care is taken to preserve the anonymity of all patients attending the clinic, their names are entered in a confidential register and they are subsequently known only by number. No information is given to anyone about the patient's condition without her permission.

Since the advent of penicillin, venereal diseases have become much less of a medical problem but the social one remains. The wide availability of 'the pill' gives good protection against unwanted pregnancy but does nothing to protect from these diseases, which can only increase with freer sexual behaviour. However, it is very important for the nurse not to be judgemental in her attitude towards patients with venereal disease, because her role is to encourage the right treatment. Patients will easily be discouraged from attending the clinic if they feel that they have to endure moral teaching. They must therefore be welcomed and accepted as they are. Similarly, patients should not be kept waiting for too long in the clinic, because they may leave unseen, especially if they are apprehensive. Their history should be taken in a private room, preferably by the doctor alone, who will not probe too deeply on the first attendance.

Patients with venereal disease usually have some suspicion of the nature of their condition before they attend the clinic, but occasionally a woman has no idea of the origin of her complaint and may attend a gynaecological outpatient department complaining of such conditions as vaginal discharge or Bartholin's abscess. It may be that she is attending an antenatal clinic and either her routine blood test or the presence of a vaginal discharge leads to further investigation. Any unmarried mother who wishes to live in a mother-and-baby home usually requires a certificate showing she is free from venereal infection.

Because venereal disease is transmitted by sexual intercourse, it is important to treat the partner whenever possible. The clinic staff and social worker in particular have a responsibility to trace contacts and persuade them to attend for examination and treatment if necessary. Many hours are spent in this task, with very little reward. Information about contacts is often misleading and unreliable and leads to false trails.

SYPHILIS

Syphilis is caused by the *Treponema pallidum*, a spiral micro-organism, and it occurs in three stages.

Primary stage

A sore, or chancre, appears about a month after infection (Fig. 23.1). This sore is the site at which the treponema entered the body, usually on the vulva or cervix, but oral

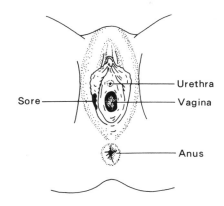

Fig. 23.1 Vulva showing primary syphilitic sore of the labium minus.

lesions may result from kissing and digital lesions from handling open sores. For this reason medical and nursing staff should wear disposable gloves whenever carrying out treatment for a patient, because of the high risk of infection.

Any lesions seen in the obstetric or gynaecological department should be investigated. The typical chancre begins as a small reddish papule which breaks down leaving a shallow ulcer about 1 cm in diameter. The female patient, who is unable to see the sore, is unaware of it as it is painless. The organisms soon penetrate into the lymphatics, and the inguinal glands become markedly enlarged. They finally reach the bloodstream about four weeks after the appearance of the chancre, when the blood may be positive to serological tests.

Secondary stage

As the primary lesion heals, the *T. pallidum* begins to spread throughout the whole body, with new signs and symptoms

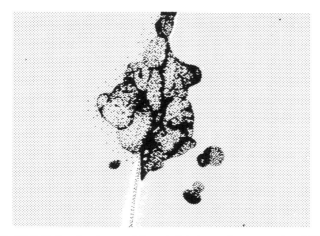

Fig. 23.2 Vulva showing condylomata lata (secondary stage of syphilis).

occurring about two months after the primary chancre. Patients may present to the gynaecologist at this stage to seek help for the condylomata lata (Fig. 23.2), which are flat-topped moist warts appearing in warm, moist areas, such as the vulva and breast flexures, and usually teeming with treponemata.

At this stage there may be mild pyrexia and general malaise, but the dominant signs are of 'snail track' ulcers on mucous membranes and of various macular and papular rashes on the skin.

The secondary stage is highly infectious, especially the mucosal surfaces. Once more it may pass unnoticed as the patient may never feel ill, the rash may be missed and other symptoms may not be urgent enough to cause the unsuspecting patient to seek advice. In a small proportion of cases the patient is obviously ill, with a widespread rash, a high pyrexia and all the symptoms of fever and toxaemia.

Tertiary stage

The tertiary stage, or late syphilis, develops at any time from 2 to 30 years after the initial infection. During this latent period the only evidence of the disorder is a positive serum test. If the early stages have passed unnoticed, the first sign may be a tertiary lesion.

In this stage lesions appear almost anywhere but particularly in the skin and subcutaneous tissues, bone, tongue, liver, aorta and the central nervous system. A localized inflammatory swelling, which is characteristically painless and known as a gumma, is formed. These swellings are firm, rubbery, greyish masses within tissue, but on the surface they are deep punched-out ulcers, regular in shape with sharp undermined edges and a 'wash leather' base. Late syphilis in particular affects the nervous system and the cardiovascular system.

Neurosyphilis Various neurological conditions may arise from a syphilitic infection.

General paralysis of the insane General paralysis of the insane occurs when the cerebral cortex is involved. There is a slow, insidious impairment of memory, judgement and intellectual faculties. As the disease progresses the patient becomes careless about her appearance, cares little for social conventions and is eventually admitted to a psychiatric hospital.

Tabes dorsalis (locomotor ataxia) Tabes dorsalis results from the degeneration of sensory fibres in the posterior root columns, leading to ataxic gait and widespread incoordination of limb movement. There are also associated shooting pains in the limbs and viscera, which may simulate an acute abdominal emergency. Trophic changes develop, giving rise to painless ulcers on the soles of the feet and joint changes (Charcot's joints).

Cardiovascular syphilis Syphilis results in elastic tissue being replaced by fibrous tissue and leads to scarring around the openings of the coronary arteries and weakening of the aortic wall.

The conditions arising are: *aortic incompetence, angina pectoris* due to *coronary stenosis, aortitis* and *aortic aneurysm.*

Diagnosis

Diagnosis may be confirmed by demonstrating the presence of the *Treponema pallidum* in exudate obtained from a chancre and examined by 'dark ground' illumination under a microscope.

Serological tests The following serological tests may be used. The first group are non-specific to syphilis, that is, they will give a positive reaction if any treponemata are present and not only *T. pallidum*. False positives sometimes follow a severe cold, glandular fever or vaccination.

Non-specific tests
   Wassermann test (WR)
   Cardiolipin Wassermann test (CWR)
   Kahn test
   Price precipitation test (PPT)
   Venereal Disease Reference Laboratory slide test (VDRL)
   Reiter protein complement-fixation test (RPCFT)

Specific tests (for syphilis only)
   Treponema pallidum immobilization test (TPI)
   (This takes 10 to 14 days and only four laboratories in this country are equipped to do this.)
   Fluorescent treponemal antibody test (FTA)
   (Easier and quicker to do.)

A selection of the non-specific tests is carried out; if these produce a positive reaction, the tests are repeated one month later. If it was a false positive, the titre gradually falls, if inconclusive then a specific test will have to be resorted to.

The exception is the pregnant woman—one cannot afford to wait a month or more because of damage to the fetus.

Treatment

Since 1944 the treatment of syphilis has been with penicillin, the patient being non-infectious in 24 hours. The most usual preparations are benzanthine penicillin (Penidural) long-acting 1.2 mega units twice weekly for six doses or procaine aluminium monostearate (PAM) 600 000 units daily for 14 days. If patients are sensitive to penicillin, aureomycin or tetracycline can be used.

In late visceral syphilis, such as cardiovascular or neuro-syphilis, the total dose of penicillin would be much larger than for early cases. Some physicians recommend preceding this with potassium iodide on account of its ability to facilitate the absorption of gummatous tissue.

After treatment has been completed, the patient must be kept under observation, routine blood tests are repeated at intervals over the next two years. On occasions a lumbar puncture and examination of the cerebrospinal fluid may also be required. If patients are treated very early, then blood tests may never be positive, or will rapidly become negative. If treated later it may take up to ten years to become negative, and those treated in the tertiary stage may remain positive for the rest of their lives. It is important when encountering positive tests to inquire whether the patient has been treated and been discharged.

CONGENITAL SYPHILIS

Syphilis may be contracted from an infected mother by the fetus in utero. After the placenta is formed, at about the tenth week, the treponemata may pass from the maternal capillaries into the fetal blood supply. This condition is rare as serological tests in the antenatal clinic have enabled prompt treatment to be given to the mother. The main danger occurs when she contracts the disease late in pregnancy after the tests have been carried out. The longer the period elapsing between infection and conception, the less likelihood there will be of an affected baby.

Clinical features
The severely affected fetus will die, which may result in an abortion or stillborn infant. In less severe cases symptoms may develop in the first three to four weeks of life. The baby may appear healthy at birth, but soon begins to lose weight and fails to thrive. There may be a widespread rash, often worse on the hands and soles of the feet, with sores around the anus like the condylomata seen in the adult. The baby has 'snuffles' and a bloodstained nasal discharge. These are due to osteitis of the nasal bones, which accounts for the saddleback nose and characteristic 'dish-shaped' face. Rhagades, or radiating scars, develop at the corners of the mouth, where skin and mucosa meet. Enlargement of the liver and spleen occurs and jaundice sometimes develops.

On occasions, congenital syphilis does not manifest itself until school age or later when interstitial keratitis leading to blindness, progressive nerve deafness and notched incisors in the second dentition (Hutchinson's teeth) occur. Congenital neurosyphilis is rare, but general paralysis of the insane can occur.

Diagnosis
Serological tests should be made on the cord blood but are of no significance unless the titre is higher than the mother's, or it is rising significantly when repeated.

Treatment
Treatment consists of penidural long-acting and procaine aluminium monostearate, as for the adult, with dosage appropriate to the age and weight of the baby.

GONORRHOEA

Gonorrhoea causes genital infection in the adult, which may consequently cause infertility because the postinfection adhesions obstruct the uterine tube in the female, or the vas deferens in the male. Gonorrhoea also causes vulvovaginitis in children and ophthalmia neonatorum in the newborn.

Early diagnosis and treatment are difficult because symptoms are often mild or absent. Often, any symptoms which do present are not associated in the patient's mind with the possibility of gonorrhoea because the incubation period is two weeks in the female (only two to five days in the male).

The causative organism is the *Neisseria gonorrhoeae*, a bean-shaped diplococcus that is found in pairs enclosed in a pus cell. The gonococcus lives and thrives on mucous membrane, and very quickly dies when removed from the human body unless the article on which it is placed is kept warm and moist. The infection is conveyed by direct contact with discharge containing the gonococci: almost always by sexual intercourse, but occasionally it may be contracted from discharge on linen or on the hands. As the organisms are harboured in the cervical glands and Skene's ducts, the patient may become infectious at intervals.

Signs and symptoms

The organism attacks the mucosa of the urethra first, causing urethritis, and then the Bartholin's gland, causing Bartholinitis. The vagina itself is not invaded but the infection spreads via the lymphatics to the cervix and uterine tubes. A patient who notices the symptoms in the acute phase gives a history of urinary frequency and dysuria, swelling and tenderness of the Bartholin's gland, and vaginal discharge. Sometimes she becomes aware of the infection when it has progressed to salpingitis, or chronic pelvic inflammatory disease, or occasionally she may develop pelvic peritonitis.

On examination, the urethra, Skene's ducts and Bartholin's ducts will usually exude pus when they are 'milked'. The cervix, which is the main reservoir of infection, appears red and inflamed, and at the external os is a thin, greenish-white discharge. A swab is taken from each area where the discharge can be seen, and must either be plated immediately or placed into Stuart's transport medium, because it is so sensitive to heat and drying. Investigations are also carried out for signs of other infection such as trichomonas, monilia, and chlamydia, and a blood test is sent for syphylis which may have been acquired at the same time.

After the examination, the nurse must be particularly careful that all instruments or gloves are disposed of carefully.

Diagnosis

A cervical smear may be examined under the microscope for quick identification, but differential diagnosis can only be made after a positive culture has been confirmed by the laboratory, either with Gram-staining or by immunofluorescence. In suspect cases, if negative results are obtained, the patient should be examined again. The gonococcal complement-fixation test (GCFT) becomes positive three weeks after infection, and may remain so after the patient has been successfully treated. It is of no value in the diagnosis of acute infections, but is occasionally helpful in chronic cases such as those found during investigations for infertility.

Treatment

Procaine penicillin 1.2 mega-units should be given daily for three days, although in the acute phase a single dose will often effect a cure if it is thought that patients will not reattend. The patient is non-infectious within 24 hours. Patients who are sensitive to penicillin are given large doses of oral cephaloridine, tetracycline and doxycycline. Following treatment, evidence of cure is established by examining smears and cultures for the presence of the gonococcus. These tests should be carried out at intervals, particularly following menstruation.

The patient is given advice about vulval hygiene, as for menstruation (see Chapter 2). If the discharge is profuse, she may be made more comfortable by gentle swabbing of the vulva and vagina with saline when she attends the special treatment centre.

Since the advent of penicillin, gonorrhoea has become less of a medical problem. The most severe effect is infertility, and the prospect of cure from the obstructions in the male or the female is still poor.

Ophthalmia neonatorum

If a woman has gonorrhoea when she is in labour, the eyes of the fetus may become infected as it passes through the vagina, by direct contact with the infected discharge. This may lead to blindness if it is not treated effectively. Ophthalmia neonatorum is a notifiable disease and highly contagious.

Signs Shortly after birth, there appears a profuse purulent greenish discharge, usually bilateral. The eyelids become red and oedematous.

Treatment The nurse's aims in management are twofold: to prevent cross-infection to other babies in the unit, and to administer prescribed treatment to eliminate the disease itself.

The baby must be isolated, and the minimum of staff should be involved in his care. The nurse, the mother and the doctors should wear gowns and gloves whenever attending to him. The nurse should explain to the mother how to use the gown properly, and why all this fuss is necessary—otherwise she may either inadvertently spread infection by poor techniques, or she may feel too daunted by the whole process.

This, compounded by her guilt that she caused the infection to her baby, may make her too frightened to go into the cubicle to care for and enjoy her baby, which could harm her relationship with him.

The baby should be laid in his cot with the most severely affected eye downwards, so that the discharge will run on to the sheet and not into the other eye. Every contaminated article, swabs, gowns, baby gowns and cot sheet, is a potential hazard; wherever feasible, disposable items should be used and burned as soon as possible.

A swab is taken for culture, and the eyes then carefully swabbed and penicillin eye drops 100 000 units in 1 ml instilled. One drop is instilled into each eye every ten minutes for an hour, if the eyes are severely infected, and the intervals between the instillations are then progressively increased until in a few hours one drop is being instilled every three hours. Systemic penicillin should also be given. The nurse must be very delicate in her touch when opening the eyelids so as not to increase the oedema. The eye should be cured within 24 hours.

Vulvovaginitis

The gonococcus may cause vulvovaginitis in children when it is transmitted via contaminated towels, bed linen or sometimes sleeping with an infected adult.

Signs The onset is usually sudden, and from the beginning there is a thick, yellow, purulent vaginal discharge, which may at times be bloodstained. There is pain and tenderness on micturition and the vulva is red and swollen, all of which may be distressing to a little girl or she may feel ashamed and confused.

Treatment A single dose of penicillin should clear the infection in 48 hours. If signs of infection persist, the possibility of reinfection or some other cause of the vulvo-vaginitis should be considered (page 265).

Education of the child and of her parents is important at this time. Her parents should be helped to understand how the infection can be transmitted to her, and it may be possible to advise them tactfully, about general hygiene and especially vulval toilet.

CHANCROID (SOFT SORE)

Chancroid, or soft sore, is a genital ulcer, a local condition which may be accompanied by lymphadenopathy but which does not cause constitutional symptoms; neither can it be transmitted to the fetus. It is highly contagious and commences within a week of intercourse with an infected male. It is a painful condition so patients normally seek help from the doctor or special clinic.

Diagnosis

Diagnosis is difficult because the Gram-negative bacillus, *Haemophilus ducreyi*, is difficult to culture and identify. The patient gives a history of one or more pustules which appeared on the vulva and vagina before breaking down and leaving multiple shallow ulcers. On examination, the ulcers have ragged edges and soft yellow irregular bases. The inguinal glands may be enlarged and tender and, later, abscesses may form.

Other venereal disease may also be present and these must be excluded.

Treatment

Chancroid responds to treatment with sulphonamides, streptomycin, choramphenicol and chlortetracycline: the effectiveness of these preparations is diagnostic, if culture of the organism was impossible.

Pain may be relieved by gently bathing the vulval area with soothing warm lotion, and with analgesics. Occasionally, it is necessary to aspirate or incise an inguinal abscess. If the patient is admitted to hospital, she is nursed in bed with barrier precautions, to prevent spread of the infection. These precautions should not, however, prevent the nurse from going in to the patient's room frequently to chat to her and comfort her, for isolation simply compounds the patient's feeling of being socially isolated as she has 'VD'.

For herpes genitalis and AIDS, see Appendix, p. 361.

FURTHER READING

PARKER. M.J. & STUCKE. V.S. (1982) *Microbiology for Nurses*, 6th ed., London: Baillière Tindall.

24 Disorders of the Cervix

INFLAMMATION OF THE CERVIX

Cervical erosion (Fig. 24.1)

Cervical erosion is an overgrowth of columnar epithelium from the cervical canal, replacing the squamous epithelium which is normally present around the external os. There may be no symptoms, but sometimes it causes postcoital bleeding. The condition is often diagnosed at routine examination, for

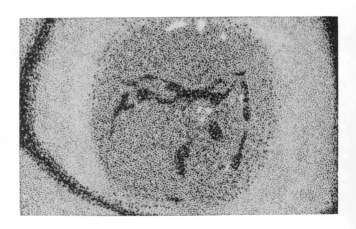

Fig. 24.1 Cervical erosion.

example at ante- or postnatal clinics, or at the family planning clinic, whenever the cervix is viewed at examination.

Treatment Cervical erosion is usually treated by cryosurgery or cauterization. A Papanicolaou's smear is always taken prior to this, to ensure that there is no malignant change.

Cryosurgery This is effective in treating mild erosion through the use of extreme cold. A probe is introduced to the cervical canal and the temperature reduced to about $-50°C$. The nurse's role is to remain beside the patient, who is fully alert but usually rather apprehensive. The treatment is almost painless and takes only a few minutes. The patient should be warned in advance that she will probably have a watery discharge for about two weeks, during which time she should avoid coitus.

Diathermy Diathermy is indicated in more extensive lesions, and is effective in destroying infected tissue by intense heat. The treatment is carried out under general anaesthesia. After the operation, burnt tissue will slough off over a fortnight causing a slightly offensive discharge, but the raw area will gradually re-epithelialize.

Cervicitis

Cervicitis is an infection of the cervix, often following an erosion. As with any inflammatory condition, cervicitis can be acute or chronic, although acute cervicitis is rare and is usually caused by the gonococcus. Chronic cervicitis is more common, though symptoms are mild. The patient may give a history of a yellow mucoid discharge which does not cause soreness or irritation of the vulva. On examination, the cervix appears red, swollen and granular, and occasionally it becomes ulcerated.

Treatment The treatment is the same as for cervical erosion.

Ectropion

Ectropion is an erosion or infection in a lacerated or gaping cervix where the columnar epithelium is exposed and becomes infected. Treatment is by cauterization or excision of the cervical lips (trachelorrhaphy).

NEW GROWTH OF THE CERVIX

Cervical polyps (Fig. 24.2)

Polyps are soft, gelatinous, pedunculated growths, which may be single or multiple and often occur following chronic cervicitis. Some may present through the external os and these are liable to ulcerate.

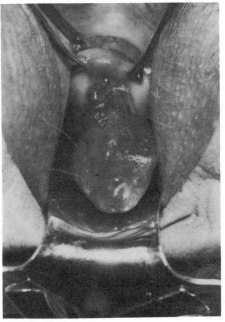

Fig. 24.2 Cervical polyp.

Treatment Polyps, being one cause of irregular bleeding, should always be removed for examination although malignancy is unlikely.

Treatment of cervical erosion, ectropion and polyps is always combined with a dilatation and curettage, as the presumption that these minor factors constitute the whole answer to the patient's history of irregular bleeding would amount to neligence in a court of law today. Malignancy must always be considered.

Carcinoma of the cervix

Carcinoma of the uterus (that is, the uterine body and the cervix) accounts for 4% of all deaths in England; 3500 women die each year from this cause and 2.7% are due to carcinoma of the cervix. Carcinoma of the cervix is twice as common as carcinoma of the uterine body. It occurs more often in women under the age of 35 years and 95% have had at least one child. It appears to be related to the standard of hygiene, the Jewish race is less susceptible than other races, contributed to in part by ritual circumcision.

The incidence in this country has lowered since health education has made women (and doctors) more open to the need for routine smear tests, and also since care has improved in family planning clinics, maternity clinics, and 'well-woman' clinics.

The site of the lesion is the squamocolumnar junction. The carcinoma grows rapidly and infiltrates the parametrium. Most cervical cancers are of the squamous cell type.

The prognosis varies according to the stage the carcinoma has reached when the patient is first seen by a doctor. Surgeons divide the degree of growth into various stages according to the extent of the growth (Fig. 24.3).

Stage O. Carcinoma *in situ*—pre-invasive.
Stage I. Direct spread, growth limited to the cervix.
Stage II. Direct spread to the fornices, parametrium and

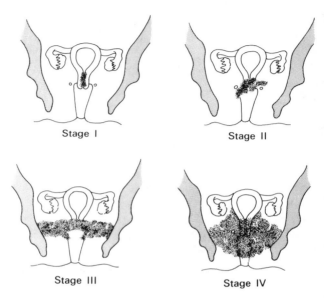

Fig. 24.3 Carcinoma of the cervix.

upper vagina; it has not reached the pelvic wall or the lower third of the vagina.

Stage III. Direct and lymphatic spread. The growth has reached the pelvic walls, body of the uterus, lower third of the vagina and pelvic lymph nodes.

Stage IV. Direct, lymphatic and blood-borne spread. The growth involves the rectum, bladder and extends outside the pelvis.

Prognosis If untreated, 90% die within three years. The five-year survival rate after treatment is:

Stage O   95–100 per cent.
Stage I   65–85 per cent.
Stage II   50–75 per cent.

Stage III 30–35 per cent.
Stage IV 8–10 per cent.

These figures speak for themselves and show how vital it is that women should seek advice early.

Tests for carcinoma of the cervix

Smear test Cervical cytology is gradually changing the picture of carcinoma of the cervix because the simple smear test reveals early histological changes which are not detected clinically. If it were possible to screen the entire population frequently enough, the disease could be virtually eliminated.

All cervices shed their most superficial layer of squamous cells into the vagina and new cells are produced from the deeper layers. It is possible, by means of an Ayre spatula (see Fig. 20.9), to pick up these cells in mucus taken from the cervix and posterior vaginal vault. This is smeared on a glass slide and immediately immersed in a solution of alcohol and ether. After staining with Papanicolaou's stain it is possible to differentiate cells which are normal, dysplastic, and malignant. Whenever the result is not normal, the smear test should be repeated and, if still abnormal, colposcopy is indicated.

Colposcopy Colposcopy means binocular inspection of the cervix at up to 20 times magnification. The doctor can view the squamocolumnar junction, where carcinoma usually commences, and his diagnosis may be made easier by using the Schiller's test or by a punch biopsy taken at the time of colposcopy.

For Schiller's test, the cervix and upper vagina are painted with a solution of iodine. Normal epithelium stains brown because it contains glycogen, but abnormal tissues do not take up the stain. This helps to identify areas for a biopsy.

A punch biopsy taken at the time of colposcopy will avoid the trauma and morbidity of a cone biopsy, which is especially important amongst young women.

Colposcopy is usually carried out in the gynaecological outpatient department, the patient being fully alert. She has special needs for reassurance, not only during an uncomfortable procedure in an embarrassing position, but more specifically she is very anxious to hear the diagnosis from what the doctor sees. In almost every patient's mind during the procedure is the idea that she may be told she has cancer. The nurse is in the privileged position of being with the patient at this important stage, and she should not undertake this duty lightly.

Biopsy Biopsy is rarely necessary for confirmation of the diagnosis since this is known from the smear test and colposcopy.

Nursing care of a patient having a cone biopsy is described later in this chapter.

Dysplasia Cervical cell dysplasia is thought to be a precursor to carcinoma *in situ*. Growth of the epithelium is seen to be disordered at histological examination, and using Schiller's test the dysplastic area does not stain brown. Treatment is as foı carcinoma *in situ*.

Carcinoma in situ There is an abrupt change in the histological appearance from the normal squamous epithelium to the abnormal area. In the absence of invasion, the lesion is designated carcinoma *in situ*, and is found in 4 per 1000 otherwise normal women between the ages of 28 and 65 years. Premalignant dysplasia is found in 12–14 women per 1000 screened. There is little doubt that nearly all these cases will develop into an invasive carcinoma at an average time interval of ten years.

When a diagnosis of carcinoma *in situ* has been made, treatment may be conservative or radical (see page 296). When the treatment is conservative, careful follow up by repeated smears must be undertaken to detect first signs of possible progression to invasive carcinoma.

Invasive carcinoma of the cervix Once the carcinoma has begun to spread, the chances of cure are diminished with each day that passes. The signs and symptoms increase as more structures become involved.

Patients in the early stages will complain of intermenstrual or postmenopausal bleeding which occurs because the surface of the growth breaks down. Initially this may be very slight and results from some minor trauma such as intercourse. Later, as the ulcerated cervix becomes infected, there will be a watery, bloodstained, offensive vaginal discharge. Pain is usually a late symptom because the cervix is relatively insensitive and pain is not felt until the growth has invaded the surrounding pelvic tissues. Finally, there is a deterioration in general health, loss of weight, weakness and severe anaemia.

As the growth spreads and destroys other structures, additional symptoms appear. Spread along the lymphatics causes blockage and the reabsorption of tissue fluid is interfered with, oedema and ascites appear. Pressure on the blood vessels impeding venous return causes varicose veins. As the bladder wall is involved frequency of micturition and haematuria occur and as more tissue is destroyed vesico-vaginal fistulae and incontinence of urine follow. Spread towards the rectum may also result in fistulae, and finally the ureters become involved, with renal failure and uraemia.

Death usually occurs from general exhaustion, uraemia or the effect of metastases. Occasionally haemorrhage occurs if a large blood vessel is eroded.

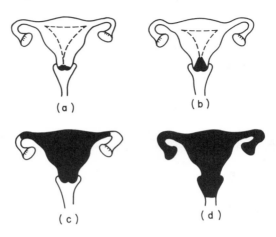

Fig. 24.4 Area of tissue removed in carcinoma of the cervix.
    (a): Ring biopsy
    (b): Cone biopsy
    (c): Simple hysterectomy
    (d): Radical surgery

Treatment Carcinoma of the cervix may be treated by surgery or radiotherapy, or a combination of both methods.

TREATMENT OF CARCINOMA BY SURGERY

Ring biopsy (Fig. 24.4(a))

Ring biopsy is the excision of the squamocolumnar junction, leaving the external os intact. This is the most conservative treatment, performed in cases of mild dysplasia when the patient is very anxious to preserve fertility. Cervical smears must be examined at least every year after a ring biopsy.

Cone biopsy (Fig. 24.4(b))

Cone biopsy is the removal of a cone-shaped area of tissue around the external os. This operation is preferred when the smear showed dysplastic or malignant cells, because it does not exclude future pregnancy yet it can eliminate carcinoma *in situ*. The biopsy allows a comprehensive diagnostic histological examination to detect invasive carcinoma which, if present, will require more radical treatment.

Conization is followed by cautery to the complete cervical ring. Postoperatively there is a likelihood of secondary haemorrhage. Prophylactic antibiotics may be given, or the patient kept in hospital under observation until after the tenth postoperative day.

The patient should be told about the morbidity from cone biopsy. Fertility may be impaired if all mucus-secreting glands are removed, or cervical incompetence may make the patient prone to abortion or premature labour. Cervical smears must be rechecked every year after a cone biopsy.

Simple hysterectomy (Fig. 24.4(c))

Simple hysterectomy is required when cone biopsy has revealed early stages of invasion or when the patient has completed her family. The nursing care of a patient having hysterectomy is described in Chapter 18.

Radical surgery (Fig. 24.4(d))

Radical surgery is indicated in invasive carcinoma, the extent of surgery being dependent upon the stage of the disease. Wertheim's hysterectomy, which includes removal of the uterus, ovaries, upper part of the vagina and much of the pelvic tissue, is adequate in most cases. This may be followed by radiotherapy if there has been lymphatic spread. In more advanced cases, extensive surgery is done, such as synchronous combined hysterocolpectomy when in addition to the above the vagina is removed; or pelvic extenteration which may include removing the bladder or rectum or both, with the transplanting of the ureters and the raising of a colostomy.

These latter extensive operations are necessary less frequently since earlier diagnosis has led to earlier treatment.

TREATMENT OF CARCINOMA BY RADIOTHERAPY

Treatment by radium or caesium

Radium is very valuable and widely used in the treatment for carcinoma of the cervix, the cure rate being as high as that achieved by surgery. Because of its rarity and value it has been replaced in many departments by caesium. The methods of treatment are identical. There are various methods of inserting radium.

Stockholm technique One tube of 50 mg of radium is inserted into the uterus and two boxes each containing 35 mg are inserted into the vault of the vagina (Fig. 24.5). Three such applications of radium are given, each insertion being

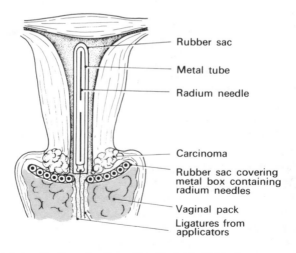

Fig. 24.5 Application of radium (Stockholm technique).

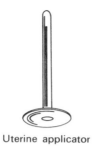

Uterine applicator

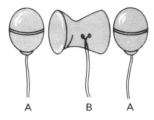

A   B   A

Fig. 24.6 Application of radium (Manchester technique).

for 22 hours; 7 days elapsing between the first and second and 14 between the second and third treatments.

Manchester technique One tube of 20 to 35 mg of radium is inserted into the uterus and two ovoids containing 20 to 25 mg placed in the fornices, spacers are used to keep them apart (Fig. 24.6). Two applications of radium are given, each insertion being for 72 hours, 3 days elapsing between each treatment. The length of treatment and number of insertions may vary, depending on the extent of the growth. In some instances application of radium is followed by external radiation of the pelvis from super-voltage machines.

Preparation of the patient The consultant and radiotherapist between them agree upon the dose to be given, which will vary with individual patients. The procedure is carefully explained to the patient, as following treatment she will experience changes associated with the menopause, if she has not already passed through this phase. Consideration is given to the position of the bed she will occupy so that too many people do not come in close contact with her for any length of time during the course of treatment. Nursing staff should wear radiation dose meters.

Vaginal douches may be given to help to minimize infection (page 221), and the rectum should be empty when the patient goes to theatre. The patient is prepared for a general anaesthetic.

Procedure The radium is inserted and the vagina carefully packed to hold it in position and to prevent excessive exposure to the bladder and rectum, since these structures, particularly the rectal wall, are easily damaged by quite small amounts of radiation. An x-ray of the pelvis is taken following insertion to ensure the radium is in the correct position. Strings from the applicators are fixed to the thigh.

On return to the ward the patient is cared for as would be any unconscious patient. A self-retaining catheter will be in position in the bladder and this is connected to a sterile bag and tubing. The ward sister signs a receipt for the radium and a card is attached to the patient's bed to denote that she has radium in position.

Care of the patient with radium implant The main aim in caring for this patient is to prevent the radium from becoming displaced, thereby possibly damaging the walls of the bladder or rectum. The vaginal pack is inserted in order to prevent displacement, but nursing care is also important because if the patient is kept as comfortable as possible she will not move excessively. The patient must stay in bed and may be nursed in the position which is most comfortable, usually semi-recumbent. If the radium is left in position for only 22 hours, it is practicable to maintain the patient's comfort and hygiene simply by washing her face and hands only, and tidying the bed. Full toilet and bed making can be carried out as soon as the radium has been removed. If, however, it is to be retained for a longer period, bed bathing and bed making must be carried out. The self-retaining catheter ensures that the bladder does not become distended and prevents the patient from having to move to get on and off bed pans. Perineal toilet is not required until the vaginal pack has been removed.

Careful four-hourly observations of the patient's temperature, pulse and respirations must be made. Any sudden rise in temperature must be reported at once since radium may aggravate latent infection; in which case it may have to be removed.

Radium insertion can be a life-saving measure but can also be dangerous if not handled correctly. At least twice a day a check should be made to see the pack and strings are in place. If wished, extra precautions can be taken to ensure that the radium cannot be lost and thus endanger other people. Special containers for rubbish and soiled linen are provided, which are not emptied until the radium has been removed and checked as correct; this prevents the possibility of radium being thrown away accidentally.

Removal of radium Radium is removed in the ward. An hour beforehand the patient is given an analgesic such as pethidine 100 mg, to enable her to relax during the procedure. The requirements include a sterile dressing trolley with a pair of long-handled radium forceps, the lead radium container, a large receiver for the vaginal pack and rubber gloves for the nurse.

The patient lies in the dorsal position, the vulva is swabbed and dried and the catheter withdrawn. The pack is then removed into the large receiver lying between the patient's legs. The strings are unfastened, and with the long-handled forceps each applicator is removed, rinsed in a bowl of water and placed in the lead container. The patient is made comfortable and the radium is returned to the radiotherapy department, where it is checked and signed for. If correct, the special containers may now be emptied.

Further treatments take place at the prescribed intervals, and in the same manner. In the meantime the patient remains in hospital, she may be up and about and take a shower or kneel in the bath to prevent too much water entering the vagina. Throughout the treatment she will need encouragement and support from the nursing staff. She will be exceedingly anxious and will easily become exhausted. Signs of a reaction to radium such as anorexia and nausea should be observed. The patient should be encouraged to drink plenty of fluids and be given what she fancies to eat. In between treatments a high-protein diet will aid tissue repair.

Treatment by deep x-ray therapy

Irradiation of the pelvis is used to treat lymphatic glands which may have been affected by the carcinoma and is frequently carried out after radium insertion or surgery. The side-effects of this treatment are frequently unpleasant for the patient, therefore one of the nurse's main responsibilities is to encourage the patient with sympathy and understanding. The patient accepts this treatment hoping that it will cure her; very often the first thing that happens is that she feels more unwell than she did before treatment began, which naturally worries her and tends to make her feel depressed.

Care must be taken to ensure that the skin over the area being treated is not irritated in any way. Deep x-rays tend to devitalize the skin and make it prone to damage that would not normally occur. The areas back and front should not be washed with soap and water but kept dry. Starch powder may be dusted on if there is any soreness. A soft nightdress and a sorbo mattress will add much to the patient's comfort. If there is a vaginal discharge, a vulval toilet with normal saline solution or a vaginal douche (using a soft rubber catheter) may be ordered. If it is necessary for the patient to wear a vulval pad, it should be kept in position with a soft T-bandage and not a belt. Nothing should be applied to the skin without reference to the radiotherapist.

Nausea and vomiting may be very troublesome and the nurse must ensure the patient has an adequate diet. Small attractive meals, extra protein and high-calorie foods are necessary, and meals should be carefully timed with treatment, so that the patient is not expected to eat when she is feeling at her lowest. Certain drugs may reduce the nausea; pyridoxine 50 mg or promethazine theoclate (Avomine) 50 mg three times a day may be useful in these circumstances. Sometimes diarrhoea is severe, in which case all roughage should be omitted from the diet and the patient encouraged to drink adequate fluids. A mixture of kaolin and morphine 15 ml, or codeine phosphate tablets 30 mg may be given in an effort to control the diarrhoea.

During the period of treatment the patient should be encouraged to be up and about as much as her condition permits, although her need for this independence must be balanced with her need for good rest. A hypnotic may be prescribed if that is necessary to help her to sleep.

Any symptom, however trivial, should be treated seriously and reported to the doctor. Sympathetic help and encouragement must be given to the patient at all times.

The patient in terminal stage

It is obvious that some patients with carcinoma will reach the surgeon too late for treatment to be effective.

Some of the complications specific to gynaecology will be pain and an offensive vaginal discharge. Fistulae of the bladder and rectum lead to incontinence of urine and faeces, and predispose to excoriation of the skin and pressure sores. Ascites may be very marked, especially when the carcinoma spreads to the ovaries, and causes much distress and discomfort.

As with all patients in the terminal stages of inoperable carcinoma, it is the nurse who is called upon to care for a patient suffering from a hopeless complaint, and she must provide the physical and mental comfort so that the patient may die when the time comes with a dignity that is the right of every human being.

FURTHER READING

TIFFANY, R. (1981) *Cancer Nursing Update*. London: Baillière Tindall.

25 Disorders of the Uterus

CONGENITAL ABNORMALITIES

During the development of the female fetus, the uterus, uterine tubes and upper part of the vagina develop from the two Mullerian ducts which fuse to form the single uterus and vagina. Defects can occur with the fusion of these ducts: fusion may either be partly incomplete with a slight dimple in the fundus of the uterus (Fig.25.1A), or in extreme cases the Mullerian ducts may completely fail to fuse, leaving two uteri and two vaginae (Fig.25.1D).

This leads to difficulties in reproduction. Diagnosis may be confirmed by hysterosalpingogram (see Chapter 15). When no treatment can be offered, the nurse's role is to comfort the patient as best she can. Even a simple friendliness and kindly manner in clinic help to soften the blow of unwelcome news to the patient.

DISORDERS OF MENSTRUATION

The interaction of the various cycles involved in menstruation is described in Chapter 2. Disorders of menstruation are described by women subjectively, since what is normal to one woman constitutes a disorder to another. The nurse must consider carefully the different needs of each patient. A few patients will require sympathetic support from the nurse because some disorders of menstruation indicate sterility or infertility. Other patients require treatment and advice for underlying causes, such as endocrine disorder. Some patients

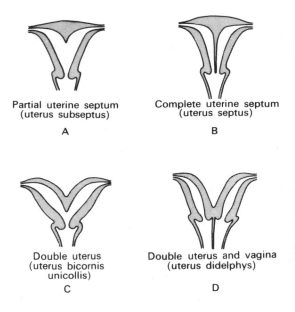

Fig. 25.1 Congenital abnormalities of the uterus and vagina.

need simple, yet easily overlooked, reassurance because the disorder is temporary and not serious.

There are four main types of disorder:

amenorrhoea—absence of menstruation

oligomenorrhoea—infrequent or scanty menstruation

dysmenorrhoea—painful menstruation

menorrhagia—excessive menstruation.

Amenorrhoea

Amenorrhoea is not a disorder in itself, but a sign of other disorder. Investigations to find the cause are carried out, such as detailed history of the condition, a general and pelvic examination, and endocrine function tests.

Amenorrhoea may be considered as primary, apparent, or secondary.

Primary amenorrhoea Primary amenorrhoea means that menstruation has never occurred. Some girls mature more slowly than others, but from the age of 17 years the condition should be investigated because after this age menstruation is less likely to start spontaneously. The hospital clinic should not only be a place where investigations, advice and treatment are given, but also where the girl can find the acceptance and understanding which she needs because she is left out of a part of womanhood. The nurse's role is to provide a mature and sympathetic setting which enables each patient to tell her problems knowing she will be understood and helped, rather than mocked as could happen at school.

Primary amenorrhoea is caused by anatomical abnormality or functional anomaly of any of the systems involved with a normal menstrual cycle (see Fig. 2.2).

The pituitary Pituitary dysfunction causes a deficiency is FSH and LH, and the amenorrhoea may be accompanied by other signs of hypopituitarism. Treatment to try to establish fertility is by artificial gonadotrophins, FSH (Pergonal) and LH (Pregnyl), as described in Chapter 15.

The ovary The menstrual cycle is disturbed only when *both* ovaries fail to develop. This is usually accompanied by underdeveloped figure and small breasts. Hormone therapy using preparations of oestrogen is effective in producing secondary female characteristics, but fertility is not normally achieved.

The uterus Menstruation cannot take place when there is no endometrium to shed, for example when the uterus has failed to develop.

Other factors Any factors which cause secondary amenorrhoea can occur before the menarche, causing primary amenorrhoea.

Apparent amenorrhoea, or cryptomenorrhoea This is not true amenorrhoea because menstruation is occurring: see Chapter 22.

Secondary amenorrhoea Secondary amenorrhoea means that menstruation ceases after it has been established for months or years. It is usually a sign of physiological and not anatomical abnormality because the patient has had normal periods. The causes of secondary amenorrhoea are as follows.

Pregnancy This commonest cause is surprisingly often overlooked when pregnancy is not expected.

Emotional upset The close anatomical and physiological relationship between the hypothalamus and pituitary can easily be affected by any psychological upset. Amenorrhoea often occurs when a woman has been bereaved, or when she is very anxious (for example about an unplanned pregnancy). Change of environment, which may be either occupation or climate, can cause menstruation to cease temporarily. Undue worry only prolongs the period of amenorrhoea.

Secondary amenorrhoea caused by these factors always rights itself; indeed, often the simple reassurance of being told so by a doctor or nurse is sufficient to precipitate menstruation.

Post-pill amenorrhoea Some women who stop taking oral contraceptives experience secondary amenorrhoea for a year or more. Treatment with clomiphene usually stimulates ovulation.

Menopause Occasionally, women have a very early menopause.

Systemic disease Any serious illness may cause menstruation to cease, or wasting disease such as tuberculosis, or the severe weight loss which accompanies anorexia nervosa.

Endocrine disorder When secondary amenorrhoea is caused by endocrine disorder, menstruation recommences when the underlying factors are treated. Common endocrine disorders are:

pituitary dysfunction—see 'Primary amenorrhoea'
hyperprolactinaemia—this may be a disorder or it may be normal, as during lactation
adrenal disease—excessive production of androgens from the adrenal inhibits menstruation
thyroid disease—hyperthyroidism or myxoedema may cause amenorrhoea.

Metropathia haemorrhagica See page 313.

Oligomenorrhoea

Oligomenorrhoea means long intervals between periods, which may occur only two or three times per year. It often heralds the onset of secondary amenorrhoea, or a premature menopause, and the causes are therefore similar. Oligomenorrhoea may also be caused by ovarian disease such as polycystic ovarian disease, tumour, or infection.

Oligomenorrhoea is often temporary, such as following the puerperium or during lactation. Ovulation sometimes occurs but fertility is usually reduced (see Chapter 15).

Dysmenorrhoea

Dysmenorrhoea is the most common gynaecological symptom; it may be primary when there is no pelvic lesion, or it may be secondary to some pathological condition. Pain which begins some time before menstruation is considered as part of the premenstrual syndrome.

Primary or spasmodic dysmenorrhoea Primary dysmenorrhoea begins in the teens, usually a year or two after the menarche. The early cycles tend to be anovular and are pain free, but it is thought that the pain occurs once ovulation begins. This pain is characterized by intermittent cramp-like spasms which, if severe, may be accompanied by vomiting, sweating and fainting. Primary dysmenorrhoea may begin a few hours before the period and seldom lasts more than 6 to 12 hours.

Management When a patient complains of pain, even if it is mild, she is seeking help from the nurse. In many instances, a hot-water bottle and mild analgesic such as paracetamol or aspirin will be sufficient. Moderate activity usually gives more relief than inactivity. She should be advised to avoid constipation just before a period is due, by taking extra fruit or a mild aperient. Mental stress will aggravate the condition and the patient may be helped if she is enabled to discuss any underlying problems.

If the dysmenorrhoea is severe, treatment with oral contraceptives is effective, although this is not always considered appropriate, for example for patients who want to avoid its side-effects or for young adolescents.

Childbirth often reduces the severity of dysmenorrhoea. Dilatation and curettage is sometimes carried out, although this entails the risk of damaging the cervix and does not always bring relief.

Presacral neurectomy interrupts pain stimuli from the pelvis, and is rarely considered in very severe cases.

Secondary or congestive dysmenorrhoea Secondary dysmenorrhoea is more common in women past teenage, usually occurring secondary to a pelvic condition such as endo-metriosis or fibroids. The pain is characterized by generalized lower abdominal pain which is probably caused by venous congestion in the pelvis. Treatment is based on the cause, but the patient will appreciate advice for any measure of relief as described for primary dysmenorrhoea (see chapter 16).

Membranous dysmenorrhoea Membranous dysmenorrhoea is a rare condition in which the whole or large parts of the endometrium are shed in one piece, which causes severe pain. Treatment is effective using the oral contraceptive pill, or the progesterone-only pill.

Premenstrual syndrome Over 50% of women are said to experience some degree of premenstrual tension. The features vary according to each patient, and arise up to ten days before the onset of menstruation and disappear as soon as the menstrual flow begins. The main symptoms described are:

mood changes, with irritability, weepiness and tension
water retention, with weigh gain of 2–3 kg
abdominal distension and breast tenderness
loss of concentration, clumsiness and lethargy
headache, backache and tiredness.

Treatment varies according to different theories as to the cause of the condition. Some patients seem to benefit from vitamin B6 (pyridoxine), and others from progestogens (such as Duphaston). The worst treatment is to tell a sufferer to pull herself together and stop bemoaning her problems. Whatever the cause of this syndrome, the patient needs comfort in whatever way that can be offered.

Menorrhagia

Menorrhagia means excessive flow of the menses; that is, either the menstrual flow is very heavy or the menstrual cycle recurs too frequently, or both. It is important to distinguish menorrhagia from metrorrhagia: the latter is not menstrual bleeding.

Some women hesitate to complain of menorrhagia, partly because they have no objective measure of what constitutes 'excessive' menstruation, and partly because they feel that they should somehow cope privately.

Of particular significance is any change in the length or frequency of the period, and an increase in the blood loss.

Causes The causes of menorrhagia are:

1. fibroids increasing the area of the uterine cavity
2. pelvic inflammation such as endometritis or salpingitis
3. endometriosis
4. adenomyosis
5. ovarian tumour
6. disturbance of the oestrogen–progesterone balance
7. thyroid dysfunction, e.g. myxoedema
8. metropathia haemorrhagica
9. certain blood disorders.

Treatment Since menorrhagia is a sign of disease, the cause must be diagnosed and treated. An examination under anaesthetic will enable the surgeon to examine the pelvis thoroughly. Curettings obtained at the same time may help to establish the diagnosis. If the cause is local, such as fibroids, myomectomy will cure the menorrhagia, but if the cause is general, treatment may be more difficult. In many cases no cause is found, although some seem to improve after a simple dilatation and curettage and others may be helped by treatment with progestogens. In severe cases where treatment is unsuccessful and the patient very debilitated, hysterectomy may be advised in older patients who have completed their family.

The patient with menorrhagia may feel generally run

down and tired, therefore she should be advised to take extra rest whenever possible, and a high-protein diet with foods rich in iron. If the chronic heavy blood loss has caused iron-deficiency anaemia, an oral iron preparation may be prescribed.

Metropathia haemorrhagica

Metropathia haemorrhagica, or cystic glandular hyperplasia, is a condition which causes menorrhagia because the endometrium becomes hyperplastic from prolonged oestrogen stimulation. It is associated with anovulation, an absence of the luteal phase of the cycle, and therefore with infertility.

The patient gives a history of grossly prolonged periods which may be heavy but are always painless. The interval between each period may be 6–12 weeks. On examination, the uterus is of normal size, but curettings show the endometrium to be thickened, vascular and non-secretory.

The aim of treatment is to restore the oestrogen–progesterone balance and improve fertility by using hormone therapy. The patient should also be given advice about her general well-being, as for menorrhagia.

Intermenstrual bleeding, or metrorrhagia

Intermenstrual bleeding is not a disorder of menstruation but is considered here because of its significance. It is bleeding from the vagina at any time other than during menstruation. It is a most important sign and must be investigated. The most serious cause is carcinoma, and the nurse should persuade any woman with irregular bleeding to consult her doctor at once. Pain is always a late symptom and because of this the other signs are often ignored until it is too late for effective treatment. Uterine carcinoma accounts for 4% of all deaths in the United Kingdom. If the cause is less serious, no harm is done by instituting early treatment.

Causes All the important causes of metrorrhagia are local lesions, not hormonal imbalance, and are therefore more easily diagnosed. The commonest causes of metrorrhagia are vaginal, cervical, or urethral conditions.

1. Vaginal conditions: trauma, ulceration from a foreign body, vaginitis and carcinoma.

2. Cervical conditions: erosion, chronic cervicitis, polyps and carcinoma.

3. Urethral conditions: urethral caruncle or carcinoma.

4. Other causes: carcinoma of the body of the uterus, endometrial polyps; ovulatory bleeding; bleeding due to the administration of hormones, particularly oral contraceptives, may all result in metrorrhagia.

Treatment The treatment of metrorrhagia is described with each causative condition.

INFLAMMATION OF THE CORPUS

Endometritis

Acute endometritis is an inflammation of the lining of the uterus, which may follow abortion, childbirth, gonorrhoea, or unsterile insertion of an intrauterine contraceptive device. The patient shows signs of infection accompanied by vaginal discharge. Treatment is usually with antibiotics.

Chronic endometritis is rare in menstruating women because the endometrium is shed regularly. It occasionally occurs after the menopause and, if the cervix has become stenosed, the infection may lead to pyometra.

Pyometra

Pyometra is a collection of pus in the uterine cavity. It can occur following childbirth or abortion when retained products or blood clot become infected, or in association with malignant disease, or as a result of cervical stenosis following operations or radiotherapy. The commonest sign is an intermittent purulent, watery or bloodstained discharge, but it may not be diagnosed until gynaecological examination. If pyometra is discovered at operation, any further surgery is postponed until the pus has been drained.

Treatment Dilatation of the cervical os allows the pyometra to drain freely per vagina, and curettage provides a specimen which can be sent for culture and the appropriate antibiotic given. On return from theatre the patient may have a rubber drainage tube inserted into the cervical canal, which will be left in situ for several days. The vulval area must be kept clean, and sterile pads should be changed frequently.

NEW GROWTH OF THE CORPUS

Endometriosis may occur in the uterine wall and elsewhere (see Chapter 28).

Endometrial polyps
There may be single or multiple polyps which arise near the fundus of the uterus. The patient usually gives a history of heavier periods accompanied by mild cramping pain from the uterus trying to expel the polyp. A vaginal discharge may occur if the polyp protrudes through the cervix. Polyps are easily removed by avulsion or by dilatation and curettage.

Fibroids (fibromyomata)
Fibroids are the commonest tumours found in women, composed of fibrous tissue and plain muscle. They are solid white tumours, usually oval or round in shape. The weight and size of fibroids vary from a tiny seed up to the size of a fetal head. They are frequently multiple, each type being named according to its location.

Intramural or interstitial fibroids (Fig. 25.2(a)) These occur within the muscle wall so when they enlarge they do not encroach on the uterine cavity. A mass may be palpated abdominally, or they may produce symptoms from pressure on other organs.

Submucous fibroids (Fig. 25.2(b)) These occur under the endometrium, giving a greater area of endometrium to shed and causing menorrhagia. Sometimes these become pedunculate and form a *fibroid polyp* (Fig. 25.3) which may be forced by uterine contractions through the external os into the vagina. It is then likely to ulcerate and cause intermittent bleeding, giving the appearance of cervical cancer.

Subserous (subperitoneal) fibroids (Fig. 25.2(c)) These occur under the peritoneum, growing away from the uterus. Their blood supply tends to become reduced, which results in degeneration. These fibroids often pedunculate and may twist.

Cervical fibroids (Fig. 25.2(d)) These occur in the cervix.

Signs and symptoms of fibroids Many women are completely unaware of having fibroids, but the nurse will see those who have developed troublesome symptoms. The patient will give a history of menorrhagia, which may result in severe anaemia. She may also complain of pressure symptoms such as backache, lower abdominal pain, constipation and urinary frequency. On examination there may be palpable abdominal tumour, and at vaginal examination the uterus is bulky and irregular. There may be leucorrhoea from the pelvic congestion.

Complications of fibroids Both menorrhagia and pressure symptoms, mentioned above, are complications of fibroids.

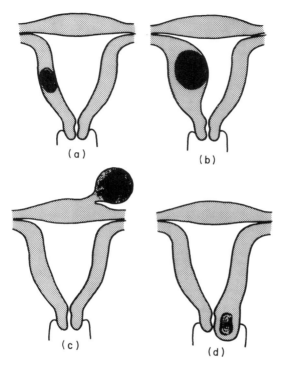

Fig. 25.2 Fibroids in the uterus. (a): **Intramural;**
(b): **Submucous;**
(c): **Pedunculated subserous;**
(d): **Cervical**

nd are by no means present in all cases. Other complications
re as follows.

Subfertility Some women with fibroids have difficulty
chieving a pregnancy or experience spontaneous abortions
ecause of the irregular-shaped uterus.

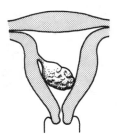

Fig. 25.3 Fibroid polyp.

Degeneration Fibroids which outgrow their blood supply may undergo degenerative changes. With red degeneration, often associated with pregnancy, there is necrosis and bleeding into the fibroid which may cause localized pain; however, surgery is rarely necessary. Other types of degeneration are hyaline, mucoid, cystic, or the fibroids may calcify or simply atrophy.

Incarceration If the fibroid is large, it can become incarcerated in the hollow of the sacrum, which may lead to constipation and pressure on the pelvic vessels, resulting in oedema, haemorrhoids and varicose veins, and during pregnancy obstruction to the descent of the fetal head.

Inversion The uterus tends to empty itself of any foreign body, and on rare occasions it tries to expel a submucous fibroid and turns itself inside out (inversion).

Torsion Polypoid fibroids may develop torsion of the pedicle, causing acute abdominal signs and symptoms.

Treatment of fibroids Small fibroids with no symptoms such as those found during routine examination, are no usually treated. Larger fibroids are treated by simple myomectomy, which means that each fibroid is shelled out and the uterus left intact. This leaves a scar on the uterus, so sometimes hysterectomy is preferable to multiple myomectomy which would leave the uterus too scarred to function normally. Hysterectomy is also indicated when there are other complications in older women.

Nursing care is described in Chapter 18. Preoperatively, if hysterectomy is a possibility, the nurse should ensure that the patient understands the doctor's explanations, and check that the necessary consent forms are signed by both husband and wife. Postoperatively, particular observation for signs of haemorrhage is necessary because of the vascularity of the area. A blood transfusion may be in progress.

Carcinoma of the body of the uterus

Carcinoma of the body of the uterus occurs much less commonly than carcinoma of the cervix, and accounts for 1% of all malignant growths. The aetiology is unknown but it is thought to be exacerbated by excessive circulating oestrogens. It tends to occur in older women between 50 and 60 years of age, and is more common in diabetic, hypertensive, and obese women.

Signs The most important sign is metrorrhagia; in the postmenopausal woman any vaginal bleeding is considered abnormal so she seeks advice quickly. She may also have an offensive vaginal discharge from an ulcerated or purulent growth. Diagnosis is made by diagnostic dilatation and curettage, the curettings showing histological changes of adenocarcinoma or (rarely) sarcoma.

Treatment Treatment is by radiotherapy or surgery, or a combination of both.

Radiotherapy often precedes surgery, and may be in the

form of an intracavity implant, or by deep x-ray therapy (see Chapter 24).

Surgery is usually confined to hysterectomy and bilateral oophorectomy. A deep cuff of vagina is often removed at the same time because of the high incidence of recurrence in the vaginal vault. Surgery is more radical if the cervix has been involved, but the myometrium seems to be an efficient barrier against spread of carcinoma.

Carcinoma of the body of the uterus is frequently a well-differentiated adenocarcinoma, slow growing and thus does not spread so rapidly. It tends to spread along the uterine tube to the pelvic lymph nodes, and later by the bloodstream to produce metastases, the commonest site being in the lungs. The poorly differentiated types invade the myometrium.

The results of treatment are good, 75% of patients being alive and free of symptoms five years later.

OPERATIONS ON THE UTERUS—VAGINAL ROUTE

Dilatation and curettage

Dilatation of the cervix and curettage of the uterus may be performed as either a diagnostic or a therapeutic procedure. It is used for diagnosis in patients with irregular or postmenopausal bleeding, or as an investigation into infertility, because curettings are sent to the pathology laboratory for histological analysis. Dilatation and curettage is curative for metropathia haemorrhagica, menorrhagia, spasmodic dysmenorrhoea and incomplete abortion to evacuate retained products of conception. The operation can also show the size, shape and position of the uterus, and the state of its cavity. Frequently it is combined with another small operation such as polypectomy or examination under anaesthetic.

This is the most common operation in a gynaecology ward which is considered by hospital staff as a 'minor' operation

The nurse should remember that going to theatre is a major event in the patient's life, however minor the operation itself may be (Fig. 25.4).

Preoperatively, in addition to routine preparation, the nurse should ensure that the date of the last menstrual period is recorded, because the surgeon will want to compare the state of the endometrium with the stage of the patient's menstrual cycle.

The operation is performed in theatre under a general or, occassionally, local anaesthetic. Graduated dilators are introduced through the cervix until the internal os will admit a sponge-holding forcep. A curette may then be passed (see Fig. 20.14) and the curettings examined.

Postoperatively, there is a vaginal loss similar to a menstrual period and sterile pads should be worn. Some patients are discharged home on the same day as the operation, and the nurse must be quite satisfied that the patient has recovered sufficiently from the anaesthetic and that vaginal loss is normal.

Culdoscopy

Culdoscopy is occasionally performed instead of a laparoscopy in order to view the pelvic viscera via an endoscope introduced through the posterior fornix. It is becoming less widely used since laparoscopy is more comprehensive (Chapter 27).

OPERATIONS ON THE UTERUS—ABDOMINAL ROUTE

Myomectomy See 'Treatment of fibroids', page 318.

Hysterectomy

The nursing care of a patient having a hysterectomy is discussed in Chapter 18. The patient's needs do not lessen after the first few postoperative days, but rather, as the

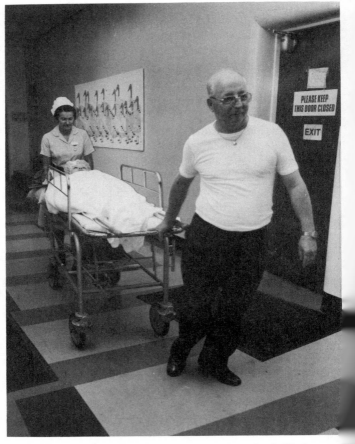

Fig. 25.4 Going to theatre is a major event in the patient's life, howeve
minor the operation itself may be.

patient's physical well-being improves, the nurse must b
increasingly astute at assessing psychosocial needs. Th
patient may mourn the loss of a part of her self, in particula

the loss of the focus of her female self. She may even grieve for the loss of an unborn (unconceived) child; or, especially in unmarried women, the end of the possibility and hope of marriage with children.

The nurse should not expect or force the patient to mourn over all these aspects, but as the patient assimilates the impact of her operation the nurse should be ready to comfort her in each area of grief as it occurs.

There are various types of hysterectomy according to the structures which are removed.

Subtotal hysterectomy This is the removal of the body of the uterus only, leaving the cervix. It is rarely performed now because carcinoma of the cervix can still occur.

Total hysterectomy (see Fig. 24.4C) This is the removal of the uterus and cervix, therefore marital relationships are unchanged although pregnancy is impossible. The ovaries will continue to function as normal until the menopause, and the ovum, when shed, will simply fall into the peritoneal cavity and die.

Total hysterectomy and bilateral salpingo-oophorectomy This is distinct from simple hysterectomy because both ovaries are removed, which artificially induces the menopause. This is especially distressing to younger women who, although they may have completed their family and may not mourn the loss of uterine function, still have to come to terms with this premature menopause. Hormone replacement therapy (HRT) is normally given, either as oral preparations or by implants of oestrogen (Oestradiol 25–100 mg) and testosterone (100 mg).

Bilateral oophorectomy is only done in more severe cases: the preservation of even a part of one ovary is sufficient to allow normal hormone function.

Wertheim's hysterectomy (radical hysterectomy) This is the removal of the uterus, uterine tubes, ovaries, upper part of the vagina, pelvic lymph nodes in the parametria and along the iliac and obturator vessels. It is an extensive operation, taking about three hours to perform, and is indicated in invasive carcinoma of the cervix.

The patient is nursed as described in Chapter 18. A radium or caesium implant may be inserted prior to the operation (see Chapter 24). After the operation a vaginal pack and an indwelling catheter may be in situ. Intravenous fluids are administered and nothing is given by mouth until bowel sounds return. Histological examination of the dissected glands will show whether or not radiotherapy is indicated after surgery.

Other abdominal operations

The following extensive operations require the full cooperation of the patient if they are to be successful, and to some, the prospect of the operation and the difficulties to follow may be more than they are prepared to face. They are fortunately done less frequently since the development of radiotherapy and chemotherapy.

Synchronous combined hysterocolpectomy This is the removal of uterus, tubes, ovaries and pelvic cellular tissues together with the vagina. It involves two surgeons, one working through the abdomen and the other working from the genital region.

Pelvic exenteration This is seldom performed unless the patient is young and otherwise fit. Even so, the outcome is disappointing and the number performed is steadily decreasing.

Anterior exenteration This is a radical hysterectomy combined with total cystectomy and transplantation of the ureters into the colon, or to an isolated ileal loop.

Posterior exenteration This is radical hysterectomy with excision of the rectum and the formation of a terminal colostomy.

Total exenteration This is radical hysterectomy with cystectomy, excision of the rectum, the formation of a terminal colostomy, and transplantation of the ureters into an ileal bladder or into the colon, a 'wet colostomy'.

26 Displacements of the Uterus

The cervix, vaginal vault and the uterus are supported by the muscles of the pelvic floor and by ligaments. If these become lax, prolapse follows. It is therefore important to learn the anatomy and physiology of these structures in order to understand the displacements of the uterus.

STRUCTURES INVOLVED IN PROLAPSE

The pelvic floor

The pelvic floor is the area of soft tissue which provides a strong support for the pelvic contents, which is especially necessary in the human because of the erect posture. It is shaped like a hammock, filling the pelvic outlet. However, it is weakened by the three structures which pierce it: the urethra, the vagina, and the rectum. Any of these three structures may be damaged or overstretched during childbirth, and if inadequate treatment is given this predisposes to genital prolapse later in life.

The deep muscles (Fig. 26.1) The deep muscles are formed mainly by the two levator ani muscles which arise from the circumference of the true pelvis and converge towards the midline, to be inserted into the perineal body, the anal canal, sacrum and coccyx. These powerful muscles are 3 to 5 mm thick. They are pierced by the rectum passing downward

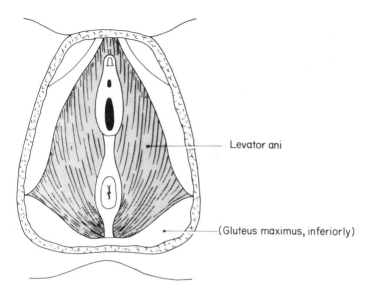

Fig. 26.1 Deep muscles of the pelvic floor.

and backwards, and the vagina and urethra passing down-wards and forwards.

The superficial muscles (Fig. 26.2) The superficial perineal muscles lie in the pelvic outlet on the undersurface of the anterior part of the levator ani muscles. They surround the anal and vaginal orifices and form the superificial half of the perineal body.

Perineal body The perineal body is a fibromuscular structure, pyramidal in shape, which lies between the lower third of the vagina and the anal canal. Fibres of the levator ani muscles form the inner half, whilst the outer half is formed from the superficial perineal muscles. It is covered with fascia and skin.

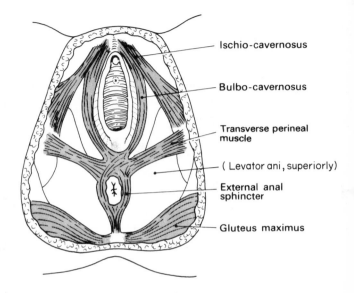

Fig. 26.2 Superficial muscles of the pelvic floor.

THE UTERINE SUPPORTS (Fig. 26.3)

Transverse cervical ligaments The transverse cervical ligaments are also known as the cardinal and Mackenrodt's ligament, radiating like a fan from the cervix and vagina to the side walls of the pelvis.

Uterosacral ligaments These run from the cervix in an upwards and backwards direction, encircling the rectum to attach to the sacrum.

Pubocervical ligaments Pubocervical ligaments run from

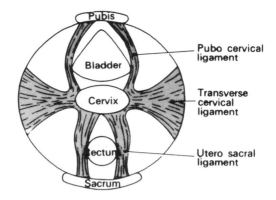

Fig. 26.3 Uterine supports seen from below.

the cervix, passing underneath the bladder to attach to the pubic bone.

Round ligaments Round ligaments originate near the fundus of the uterus, passing through the inguinal canal and anterior abdominal wall to the labia majora.

Note. The broad ligaments are folds of peritoneum and, despite their name, they are not ligaments and in no way support the uterus.

GENITAL PROLAPSE

Prolapse is the downward displacement or herniation of the uterus and/or vaginal walls. As with any hernia, two factors are necessary: a weakness in some structure (in this case the pelvic floor), and an increase in intra-abdominal pressure.

In most instances the pelvic floor is weakened as a result of obstetric trauma; prolapse is uncommon in nulliparous women. Although the actual damage to the supports has usually occurred during pregnancy and labour, many women are unaware of any abnormality until the menopause. At this time oestrogen levels fall, the uterine supports atrophy, and not infrequently there is a gain in weight and loss of muscle tone. These factors allow the pelvic organs to sag through the weakened pelvic floor and so cause symptoms. In some women a contributory factor is a constitutional weakness of the ligaments.

Intra-abdominal pressure is increased with coughing, as in chronic bronchitis, constipation, obesity, large abdominal tumours or heavy industrial work involving lifting and straining. These may all predispose to genital prolapse.

When the vaginal walls prolapse, other pelvic organs which lie adjacent to them are also displaced. Thus the terms used to describe prolapse relate to the organ behind the defective vaginal wall.

Anterior vaginal prolapse
This may occur alone but is usually secondary to uterine descent.

Cystocele There is a weakness in the upper part of the anterior vaginal wall which allows the bladder to bulge into the vagina. The swelling increases in size when coughing and it is usually accompanied by stress incontinence and recurrent cystitis.

Urethrocele The urethra bulges into the lower vaginal wall, this also predisposes to stress incontinence.

Posterior vaginal prolapse

Enterocele or vault prolapse The pouch of Douglas herniates into the upper posterior vaginal wall, and may contain small bowel and occasionally omentum.

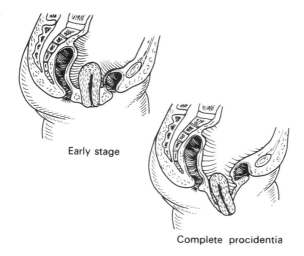

Early stage

Complete procidentia

Fig. 26.4 Prolapse of the uterus (early and complete procidentia).

Rectocele The rectum bulges into the lower posterior vaginal wall. A small rectocele may produce no symptoms but in a severe condition there may be difficulty in defaecation.

Uterine prolapse

The transverse cervical (cardinal) ligaments are weakened and the uterus descends down into the vagina (Fig. 26.4).

Three degrees are described.

First degree—the uterus has descended but the cervix has not reached the introitus.

Second degree—the uterus descends farther and the cervix protrudes from the vaginal orifice.

Third degree or procidentia—the entire uterus lies outside the vaginal orifice, the vagina being turned inside out.

Signs and symptoms The signs and symptoms of genital prolapse vary from patient to patient, according to whether the uterus, bladder or rectum is most markedly displaced. Certain symptoms are common to all.

The patient complains of a 'lump' in the vagina, or a feeling of 'something coming down'. She has a vague feeling of pressure in the lower abdomen, and possibly also backache when standing. As the descent worsens, she has increasing difficulty in sitting and walking normally.

On examination, the prolapse can be seen using Sim's speculum, unless it is very small. An offensive, bloodstained vaginal discharge may be present if the vagina, cervix or uterus is ulcerated from the friction as the cervix rubs against the vaginal walls and later on the patient's clothing.

Constipation is a particular feature of rectocele, and straining only makes the condition worse.

If there is a cystocele, the patient will probably have signs and symptoms of urinary infection, and on examination there is nearly always residual urine in the bladder. Any impingement on the urethra quickly leads to stress incontinence. For the fastidious woman, this is perhaps the most distressing symptom; any rise in intra-abdominal pressure from coughing, laughing or sneezing causes urine to leak from the bladder. Her inability to control this causes embarrassment and insecurity, as well as the uncomfortable feeling of damp clothing.

Intravenous pyelography and a micturating cystogram may also aid the doctor in his decision as to which treatment is most suitable.

Management of prolapse

Prevention Prevention is much better than cure, and the nurse can help patients in two specific ways: by teaching exercises to be done ante- and postnatally and postoperatively, and by helping to prevent trauma during labour.

Exercises are always good to maintain good muscle tone, but they are especially important to build up pelvic floor muscles weakened by childbirth and operations. The nurse should work closely with the physiotherapist in teaching exercises specific to the pelvic floor muscles.

During labour, thorough observation and clear written records highlight any abnormalities as soon as they occur, thus helping towards prompt action in the event of prolonged labour. Great care must be taken whilst using obstetric forceps, to prevent shearing of the muscles, and although this is the doctor's remit the nurse can help by being efficient in assisting him. Fundal pressure when delivering the placenta can damage the transverse ligaments.

Palliative treatment A pessary is often sufficient to restore the uterus to its former position, depending on the patient's age, general condition and her desire for more children. Most gynaecologists favour the watch-spring pessary; this has a coiled spring incorporated in the rim, which allows it to keep its shape better than the soft rubber or plastic ring pessary which distorts readily (Fig. 26.5).

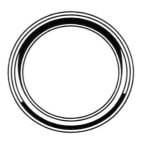

Fig. 26.5 Ring pessary.

Insertion Pessaries are not usually inserted by the nurse, but she may be required to change one. The patient should be placed in the left lateral position and the vulva then exposed. Gloves should be worn and the nurse should cleanse the area with an antiseptic lotion. The pessary is dipped in lubricant, squeezed between the thumb and fore-finger of the right hand, and with the left hand separating the labia it is slipped into the vagina and released. With two fingers she then pushes one edge until it slips into the anterior fornix, and the other into the posterior fornix. If the ring is correctly in position, the cervix should project through the ring and the uterus should be supported.

Advice The patient is told she must wash the vulva thoroughly every day, preferably using a bidet, and to return at once if she is uncomfortable. The ring will require changing every three months, which is an arduous procedure, but necessary as all rings cause some degree of vaginitis and if that is neglected ulceration may occur. Many elderly patients will require the help of the district nurse, and the necessary arrangements should be made by the hospital or general practitioner.

Surgical treatment The aim of surgery is to reconstruct the muscles and ligaments which support the bladder, rectum and uterus and to replace them in their original positions. Such a repair is the treatment of choice, and cure or relief is obtained in 95% of cases. If the patient is a young woman, further pregnancies are possible. Each operation is explained below.

OPERATIONS USED IN PROLAPSE

Anterior colporrhaphy Anterior colporrhaphy is a repair to correct a prolapse of the anterior vaginal wall, by excising a triangular-shaped area, restoring the bladder and urethra to their correct positions and reconstructing the vagina. The nurse can reassure the patient that she need not be afraid of a bowel movement because the rectum is posterior so there is no direct pressure on the (anterior) suture line.

Posterior colpoperineorrhaphy Posterior colpoperineorrhaphy is a repair to correct prolapse of the posterior vaginal wall. A triangular area of the posterior wall is removed, the rectum carefully freed from the vagina and the vaginal skin then sewn together narrowing the lumen of the vagina. The muscles of the perineal body are approximated in the midline (perineorrhaphy) and the remaining skin area sutured.

Special attention must be given to preoperative preparation of the bowel, and postoperative use of aperients.

Repair of enterocele or vaginal vault Repair of the upper posterior wall is usually undertaken as part of a Manchester repair or a posterior colporrhaphy.

Manchester repair or Fothergill's operation Manchester repair is performed when there is descent of the uterus and laxity of the vaginal walls. In this case the elongated cervix is amputated, the transverse ligaments are shortened by stitching them in front of the uterus; the operation is completed by an anterior and posterior colpoperineorrhaphy (Fig. 26.6).

The detailed nursing care of this condition is given in Chapter 18.

Vaginal hysterectomy Vaginal hysterectomy (or Mayo Ward operation) may be performed when there is a procidentia, or when uterine disease complicates a lesser degree of prolapse. The vaginal wall is divided, the uterus is pulled down, freed from ligaments, peritoneum and uterine tubes,

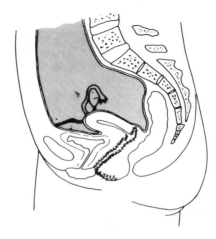

Fig. 26.6 Diagram to show extent of sutures following repair operation.

and then removed. The peritoneum is closed and the round ligament, uterine tube, ovarian ligament, transverse ligament and uterosacral ligament are attached to the vagina to form a new vaginal vault. An anterior and posterior repair is carried out to complete the operation.

Preoperatively, additional local treatment is required if the cervix reaches beyond the introitus, to reduce oedema and treat any ulceration that is present. Postoperatively, there is a higher risk of concealed haemorrhage than for repair operations because the peritoneum has been opened. The discharge following vaginal hysterectomy is usually profuse but should not be offensive.

Marshall Marchetti Kranz This is an abdominal operation for the relief of stress incontinence when vaginal operations have failed. The object of the operation is to elevate the bladder neck and the bladder itself, and so restore the normal angle between the bladder and urethra. The fascia adjacent to the urethra and bladder neck is sutured to the periosteum at the back of the symphysis pubis, causing the bladder neck to be drawn upwards and forwards. This is a relatively simple operation, the results are good and the complications few. Postoperatively bladder drainage is maintained for three to five days, after which time the patient passes urine without difficulty.

RETROVERSION

The uterus is displaced backwards into the pouch of Douglas from its normal anteflexed and anteverted position. Retroversion can be congenital or acquired.

Congenital retroversion

Congenital retroversion has no clinical significance and many women are unaware of its existence. It rarely causes symptoms except related to pregnancy (see Chapter 5).

Acquired retroversion

Acquired retroversion is mostly caused by the stretching of the uterosacral and round ligaments during pregnancy and labour and their failure to involute during the puerperium. Occasionally it is associated with infection, notably tuberculosis but also salpingo-oophoritis and endometriosis, because adhesions form and bind the uterus down into the retroverted position. This latter is called **fixed retroversion** (see Fig. 26.8 and compare with Fig. 26.7).

Diagnosis Retroversion does not usually cause symptoms in itself, although the patient may complain of symptoms which are related to the causative adhesions or infection. Diagnosis is made at vaginal examination by the position of the cervix, as illustrated in Fig. 26.8.

Occasionally, a patient will complain of backache and

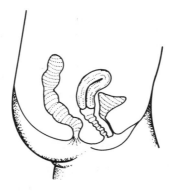

Fig. 26.7 Normal position of the uterus.

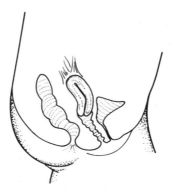

Fig. 26.8 Uterus retroverted and fixed by adhesions.

dysmenorrhoea which is relieved by the insertion of a Hodge pessary: this is helpfully diagnostic of retroversion.

Treatment Treatment may be conservative or surgical, depending on the age of the patient and the cause of the retroversion.

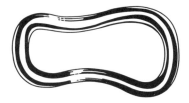

Fig. 26.9 Hodge pessary.

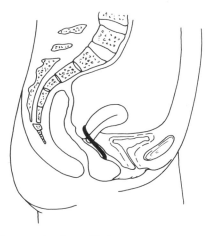

Fig. 26.10 Diagram showing a Hodge pessary in position.

Retroversion of the uterus following childbirth can be corrected by the insertion of a Hodge pessary (Figs. 26.9 and 26.10). This is inserted by a gynaecologist with the longer limb behind the uterus, and kept in position for six to eight weeks until the ligaments have become stronger. Aftercare is as for a ring pessary (page 334).

Surgical correction (ventrosuspension) may be indicated in the younger woman to restore the uterus to its natural position. Occasionally in older women, if the retroversion is caused by or complicated by other factors such as tumour in the pelvis, hysterectomy is carried out.

Ventrosuspension operation of the uterus Ventrosuspension is an operation to correct a fixed retroversion of the uterus. The round ligaments are pulled through the musculature of the abdominal wall just above the symphysis pubis and sutured to each other and to the rectus muscle, thus pulling the uterus forward and forming a sling underneath it.

Ventrosuspension has become a less traumatic operation since it can now be done via the laparoscope, but the patient still experiences the same pulling pain internally, even though the abdominal wound is much smaller. This operation does not interfere with subsequent pregnancies or labour.

Ventrosuspension of the ovaries If there is deep dyspareunia from the prolapsed ovaries, these can be elevated to their original position by plicating (pleating) sutures through the fascia.

27 Disorders of the Uterine Tubes

THE UTERINE TUBES

The uterine or fallopian tubes extend laterally from the cornua of the uterus almost to the side walls of the pelvis, they then turn backwards and downwards towards the ovaries.

Each tube is 10 to 11.5 cm in length and is divided into four parts (Fig. 27.1).

The interstitial portion, which passes through the wall of the uterus and has the narrowest lumen.
The isthmus, slightly wider than the interstitial area.
The ampulla, where it widens out.
The infundibulum, composed of a number of finger-like processes, or fimbriae, which communicate with the peritoneal cavity. One fimbria is slightly longer than the

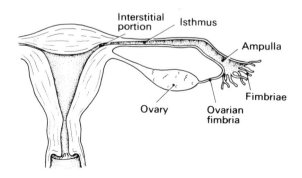

Fig. 27.1 Divisions of the uterine tube.

rest and attaches to the ovary below, it is known as the fimbria ovarica.

Structure

The uterine tube has three coats.

1. A covering of peritoneum (the broad ligament).

2. A thin muscle coat of circular and longitudinal fibres which enables it to undergo peristalsis.

3. A lining of ciliated columnar epithelium which wafts from the infundibulum towards the cornua. This lining is thrown into so many folds that the lumen is not easily seen (Fig. 27.2).

The cilia speed the ovum through the tube and the numerous folds tend to slow down its passage, thus a delicate balance is achieved. If the ovum passes too rapidly, it is not developed sufficiently to embed in the uterine wall and is lost. Conversely, if the journey is too slow it may grow too large to pass through the narrow interstitial portion resulting in a tubal pregnancy. If the cilia of both tubes are so damaged by previous infection as to block the lumen completely, the spermatozoa can never reach the ovum, so a pregnancy cannot ensue.

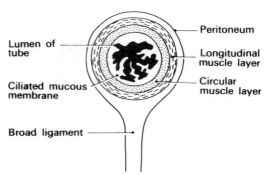

Fig. 27.2 Section through the uterine tube.

The blood supply is from the ovarian artery and uterine artery. This double blood supply is of great importance and no matter how severe an infection of the tube may be, gangrene will not occur. Venous drainage is by veins of the same name and the nerve supply is derived from the sympathetic and parasympathetic systems.

INFLAMMATION

Salpingitis

Salpingitis is inflammation of the uterine tube, and may be uni- or bilateral. In many cases the ovaries are involved and the condition is called salpingo-oophoritis. Salpingitis is a significant condition because the tubes, when patent, form a direct connection with the peritoneal cavity so any infection can spread rapidly to pelvic peritonitis; furthermore, once chronic salpingitis is established, infertility often follows.

The tube becomes tense, red and swollen and the lumen is filled with pus. The fimbriated end may be blocked by adhesions and if the interstitial end becomes swollen with oedema, pus is trapped in the tube which distends more and more: this is now a *pyosalpinx*.

Spread may occur locally causing an ovarian, tubo-ovarian or pelvic abscess; adhesions form and bind the uterus and its appendages to the omentum and gut. The condition may resolve completely but often there is fibrosis which leads to blocking of the lumen of the tube and infertility: this shows on a hysterosalpingogram (see Chapter 15).

Causes The causative organisms are gonococci, staphylococci, streptococci, pneumococci and coliforms.

Infection may be ascending (e.g. gonorrhoea); or by direct contact with an inflamed structure (e.g. appendicitis); or blood borne (e.g. tuberculosis). Some 60–75% of infections

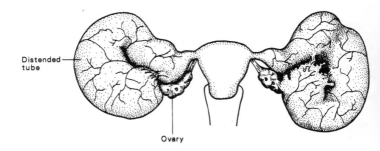

Distended
tube

Ovary

Fig. 27.3 Bilateral hydrosalpinx.

are caused by the gonococcus, and the remainder follow appendicectomy and puerperal or postabortal infection.

Signs and symptoms The patient complains of lower abdominal pain, often bilateral and associated with malaise, headache and pyrexia. Frequency of micturition and dysuria are common, giving a confusing picture of urinary infection. Vomiting is unusual. On examination, there is often a purulent vaginal discharge, in which case a high vaginal swab is taken to culture the organism. A midstream specimen of urine is also sent to the laboratory.

Occasionally, laparoscopy may be indicated to differentiate the diagnosis from appendicitis or ectopic gestation (see Chapter 5).

Treatment The aims of management are to relieve symptoms and to cure the infection promptly so as to prevent the complications of chronic salpingitis arising.

The patient should be admitted to hospital, confined to bed and carefully observed. Pain may we relieved by a well covered hot-water bottle or electric pad over the abdomen and analgesics such as paracetamol, codeine or pethidin may be given. Dysuria may be relieved by keeping the urin alkaline with potassium citrate mixture. The patient should be supported comfortably with pillows, and her toilet needs attended to. Special care must be given to the vulval area while the discharge is profuse. The fluid intake should be 3000 ml, and light attractive meals will be given. The temperature, pulse and respiratory rate are recorded four-hourly, and fluid intake and urinary output measured daily.

Antibiotics are prescribed after the high vaginal swab has been taken. As with any inflammation, rest is very important, so the nurse should ensure that hospital routine does not prevent this therapy.

Occasionally a pelvic abscess forms, which requires surgical drainage.

Chronic salpingitis

If the condition does not resolve, the infection becomes chronic, and gross fibrosis and thickening occur. Once the infection is chronic it is rare to identify any organism except in the case of tuberculosis.

Oedema and adhesions quickly seal off the tubes, which swell up, filling with a watery exudate: this is a hydrosalpinx (Fig. 27.3). The tube can become convoluted and densely adherent to the ovary.

Signs and symptoms The patient gives a history of repeated attacks of abdominal pain and pyrexia. This may be accompanied by general ill-health with menorrhagia, anaemia, congestive dysmenorrhoea, and backache. Deep dyspareunia, bladder irritability and infertility may also occur.

Treatment Continual pain is very wearisome to the patient, especially when accompanied by anaemia and general ill-health. The nurse can become as disheartened as the patient if the disease is not cured, but she can always bring comfort, both physically by high standards of nursing care, and also mentally by carrying out her duties with compassion and understanding.

Treatment is conservative at first, as for the acute condition, with additional measures to try to eradicate the infection completely and to re-establish better general health. In addition to bed rest and antibiotic therapy, short-wave diathermy to the pelvis if often helpful. Anaemia is corrected with iron preparations. If the patient is young and wanting a family, further investigations or treatment for infertility may be carried out as described in Chapter 15.

Surgery is often necessary if the condition does not improve with these conservative measures. An exploratory laparoscopy will usually decide the extent of damage, and the surgeon may proceed to a laparotomy to remove the tube and ovary (salpingo-oophorectomy), or to divide painful adhesions (salpingolysis). On rare occasions, when the patient is severely debilitated by recurrent infection, hysterectomy may be performed.

Tuberculous salpingitis

Although chronic in nature, this frequently responds well to treatment with antituberculous drugs without resort to surgery. It usually results from a pulmonary focus and in 60% of cases results in infertility.

NEW GROWTH

Primary carcinoma of the tube is exceedingly rare and the prognosis very poor.

Secondary carcimoma is more common and results from the extension of a primary carcinoma in the uterus (see Chapter 25).

OPERATIONS ON THE UTERINE TUBE

Salpingectomy

Salpingectomy, or the removal of a uterine tube, is performed for tubal rupture following an ectopic pregnancy, or tubal disease such as pysosalpinx or hydrosalpinx. In the former case it is an acute surgical emergency.

Salpingectomy is often combined with other operations such as oophorectomy or hysterectomy.

Salpingo-oophorectomy When the ovary is diseased it may be necessary to remove it with the tube. This operation is often preferred to a simple salpingectomy, even when the ovary is healthy, because an ovum, having no tube to pass down when shed, falls into the peritoneal cavity and could be fertilized and cause an extrauterine pregnancy.

The patient should be reassured that her hormones adjust immediately to unilateral oophorectomy, and that ovulation occurs every month as normal from the one remaining ovary.

Bilateral partial salpingectomy (sterilization) See Chapter 16.

Laparoscopy Laparoscopy is an operation to view the contents of the pelvis, and is preferable to laparotomy because it involves much less trauma. It is performed for any of three main purposes.

Diagnosis The surgeon can identify conditions such as tubal pregnancy or endometriosis, or take biopsies via a cannula.

Investigation of infertility Laparoscopic dye test (see Chapter 15).

Sterilization The tubes can be occluded by a clip or by diathermy.

The operation is performed under local or general anaesthesia. Two small incisions are made: one for the cannula through which carbon dioxide is passed so that the pelvis can be viewed, and a second for the laparoscope itself.

On return from theatre the patient is nursed flat for a few hours. She should be told of the findings before she goes home: this may be on the same day if she had a local anaesthetic. The patient should return on the appropriate day to have her sutures removed.

Operations to restore tubal patency

There are many operations for this purpose, known as tuboplasty, but they are very intricate, often requiring the use of the microscope in theatre. Results from these operations are often disappointing.

Patients in hospital having these operations need physical care as after any major operation, but they also need much encouragement because they tend to spend many hours pondering over their inability to conceive.

Salpingolysis This is an operation to divide adhesions around the outside of the tube, especially the fimbriated end. All the raw surfaces are covered with perintoneum to prevent further adhesions and the fimbriated end is left close to the ovary.

The patient usually finds immediate relief from the pain caused by adhesions and makes a rapid recovery, especially if the operation was performed via the laparoscope.

Salpingostomy Salpingostomy means making an opening into the tube and is usually carried out to restore patency in an obstruction near the fimbriated end. Several methods are used.

1. The fimbriated end and the obstruction are removed and the mucosa is turned back as a cuff over the cut edge of the tube and sutured in place.

2. The fimbriated end is slit behind and two triangular-shaped flaps are folded back and sutured along the tube.

3. An artificial opening is made in the tube proximal to the obstruction.

Tubal reimplantation When the obstruction is in the isthmus or interstitial portion, the tube is divided beyond the obstruction. The remaining tube is dissected out of the cornua and the distal end implanted into the opening.

Salpingoplasty When the obstruction is in the isthmus, the tube is divided on either side of it, the obstruction removed and the two ends anastomosed, sometimes over a polythene splint. The splints are removed some days later through the vagina.

28 Disorders of the Ovary

INFLAMMATION

Oophoritis

Oophoritis is an infection of the ovary which often accompanies an infection of the uterine tube as salpingo-oophoritis. The signs, symptoms and nursing care of this are given in Chapter 27.

Less commonly, oophoritis may occur in a young woman as a complication of mumps (similar aetiology to orchitis in the young male).

NEW GROWTH

The ovary, being a reproductive organ, possesses cells of great potential and it is not surprising that tumours of the ovary present in many different forms; some are cystic and others solid tumours occurring most commonly during the reproductive years. Signs, symptoms and complications are given on page 357, after describing the types of new growth. Most of them are benign but in the very young or the woman over 50 years they are likely to be malignant.

New growths in the ovary may be cystic or solid.

Cystic tumours

Simple serous cysts (cystadenomas) Simple cysts occur at any time during the reproductive phase but most commonly

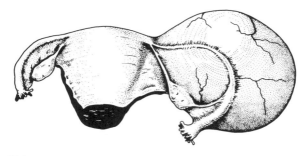

Fig. 28.1 Uterus with simple serous cyst.

between the ages of 30 and 40 years. They are often unilocular (having a single cavity), contain clear yellow fluid and are about 5 cm in size, although some are very much larger (Fig. 28.1). One-quarter to a half occur bilaterally, and some show malignant changes. They are very often asymptomatic, but should they have papillae these may grow through the cyst wall into the abdominal cavity and cause ascites.

Pseudomucinous multilocular cysts These are large, multicavity cysts containing a sticky mucinous-like material (Fig. 28.2). They occur between the ages of 30 and 50 years, are

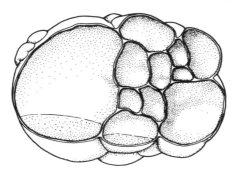

Fig. 28.2 Multilocular ovarian cyst.

rarely bilateral, rarely malignant and have papillae in 25% of cases.

Papilliferous cysts Papillae may complicate serous or pseudomucinous cysts; they are warty excrescences which grow on the cyst walls. These sometimes penetrate through into the peritoneal cavity and cause ascites. Papilliferous cysts have a greater potentiality to malignancy than cysts where papillae are absent.

Endometrioma Endometrioma are cysts which are part of a condition called *endometriosis*, in which endometrial tissue grows outside the cavity of the uterus. The cells are often present in the ovary, and bleeding corresponding to the menstrual flow takes place in them, causing an accumulation of blood. The cysts themselves contain altered blood of a dark-brown colour, hence their name 'chocolate cysts'.

Many theories exist to explain the presence of the endometrial cells outside the uterus, but it is possibly secondary to a reverse flow of menstrual loss along the uterine tube into the peritoneal cavity, carrying with it shreds of endometrium. Whatever the aetiology, it is known that the stimulus of ovarian oestrogens is necessary.

Signs and symptoms Symptoms appear in the late twenties and thirties, and are predominantly lower abdominal pain, dyspareunia and infertility. The dull aching or cramp-like pain is worst before and during menstruation. Diagnosis is confirmed at laparoscopy when the endometrioma are viewed.

Treatment Treatment is first conservative, aiming to suppress endometrial activity with hormones. Progestogen (e.g. norethisterone 5 mg daily) effectively relieve symptoms during the course of treatment, while anti-oestrogens (e.g.

danazol 400 mg daily) not only relieve symptoms but can also cause regression and allow a pregnancy.

Surgery may be necessary, depending on the severity of symptoms and the response to drugs. Endometrial tissue or cysts are removed, or occasionally a hysterectomy is indicated with or without oophorectomy.

Teratoma or dermoid cysts These bizarre tumours arouse considerable interest. They contain elements from all three germinal layers, endoderm, ectoderm and mesoderm. They are quite common, occurring between the ages of 20 and 40 years, are occasionally bilateral and almost always benign. The tumours are usualy pedunculated, smooth, round with a glistening grey surface and containing a thick sebaceous material and tangled masses of hair growing from a solid area at one end (Fig. 28.3). This solid area may contain elements of tissue found in skin, sweat glands, respiratory epithelium,

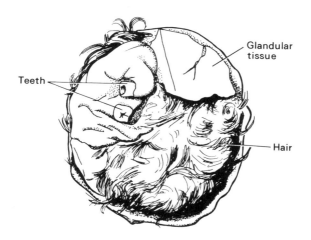

Fig. 28.3 Dermoid cyst.

salivary glands, nervous tissue and occasionally thyroid tissue which if secreting can cause thyrotoxicosis. Quite a large number contain formed teeth which often lead to their diagnosis as they are visible on a pelvic x-ray. They rarely cause symptoms unless torsion occurs, and are not uncommonly discovered during an antenatal examination.

Malignant teratoma These are compact, solid, rapidly growing tumours containing elements of germinal layers similar to the dermoid cysts. They may occur at any age but frequently the patient is young. Mesoderm predominates and there are elements of connective tissue, cartilage, fragments of bone and muscle. The prognosis is very poor.

Retention cysts
These are cysts arising from the ovarian follicles at different phases of the cycle.

Follicular cysts These result when a graafian follicle fails to rupture but continues to grow in size, and rarely exceed 3 cm in diameter. They are usually multiple and bilateral. Symptoms are rare unless the cysts are large or complicated by rupture or haemorrhage. They are often associated with endometrial hyperplasia and uterine fibroids.

Luteal cysts These develop from the corpus luteum. Symptoms are usually related to their size, but they may cause amenorrhoea followed by irregular uterine bleeding. Complications such as torsions, rupture or haemorrhage may occur.

Multiple cysts (polycystic ovarian disease) This is a condition sometimes known as Stein–Leventhal syndrome in which there is excessive production of androgens by the ovary. Many follicles develop and become cystic, bu without releasing the ovum. This causes anovulation, oligo-menorrhoea or secondary amenorrhoea, infertility, and some-times masculinization. On examination the ovary is enlarged, and at laparoscopy it is seen to have multiple follicular cysts and no corpus luteum. Treatment is difficult but occasionally a wedge resection of the ovary is performed to try to reduce ovarian activity. If appropriate, treatment may include the use of clomiphene or artificial LH (Pregnyl) to try to restore fertility (see Chapter 15).

Functioning ovarian tumours

Feminizing tumours (granulosa cell tumours) These tu-mours arise from the cortex and frequently produce steroids. In childhood they cause precocious female development and in older women, menopausal and postmenopausal bleeding. About one-third become malignant.

Masculinizing tumours (arrhenoblastoma) These tumours produce virilizing effects such as amenorrhoea, growth of facial hair, enlargment of the clitoris and deepening of the voice. One-quarter become malignant.

Patients with these tumours need kind acceptance despite their appearance, but they can be reassured that these features disappear within weeks of the removal of the tumour. Voice changes tend to be permanent.

Solid tumours

Fibroma Fibromas are innocent tumours, firm, hard and greyish white in colour composed of fibrous tissue, occurring most frequently in middle-aged women (Fig. 28.4). They may be bilateral and produce no specific symptoms. Oc-casionally they cause ascites, pleural effusion and cachexia and may be confused with carcinoma; however, these symptoms disappear when the tumour is removed.

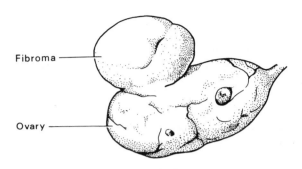

Fig. 28.4 Fibroma.

Carcinoma Carcinoma may occur in the ovaries at any time but most commonly between the ages of 40 and 60 years. Early diagnosis is important because the prognosis is poor. Carcinoma may be a primary or secondary growth.

Primary ovarian carcinoma In the majority of cases this is preceded by a benign growth and is rarely suspected until signs appear from its spread to other structures; such as abdominal distension, chronic low abdominal pain and post-menopausal bleeding.

Secondary ovarian carcinoma Metastic deposits may be from other organs such as the uterus, cervix and breast. There may also by lymphatic spread from a primary growth in the alimentary tract: in this instance the ovarian growth is known as Krukenberg's tumour.

It is important that the surgeon is certain whether this is a primary or secondary growth as this could radically affect the treatment. In the case of a secondary growth it is unlikely that surgery will be of much avail.

Signs and symptoms of new growth

Signs and symptoms often appear late in benign and malignant tumours. Many are diagnosed on palpation during a medical examination, while others are not diagnosed until complications occur.

Increasing girth The patient may be aware of increasing abdominal girth, or frequent necessity to let out the waistbands on clothing.

Pressure symptoms Pressure on the bladder may cause frequency of micturition or retention with overlow. If the cyst becomes impacted in the pelvis, constipation may result. Very large cysts may cause a feeling of heaviness in the pelvis, and predispose to oedema and varicose veins because of interference with the venous return and lymphatic drainage. Pressure on the diaphragm causes breathlessness.

Menstrual changes Amenorrhoea is uncommon even with large cysts; functional tumours, however, may alter the menstrual pattern and scanty loss may occur followed in some cases by profuse, irregular bleeding. Ovarian carcinoma may cause postmenopausal bleeding.

Pain Pain is rare in the uncomplicated tumour and is more likely to result from rupture, torsion, haemorrhage or sudden rapid distension of the cyst. Ovarian pain is a constant ache referred to the lower back, the inguinal region and inner aspect of the thigh, occasionally radiating to the vulva.

Complications of new growths

Torsion Many benign tumours, both cystic and solid, develop long pedicles, which may twist at any time. This may occur gradually, in which case the patient complains of increasing pain and tenderness, or it may twist suddenly causing severe pain. This resembles the signs of an acute abdominal condition: the patient is anxious and frightened, the pulse rapid, skin cold and clammy, and nausea and vomiting may be present. Congestion occurs because of the pressure on the blood vessels and this could result in gangrene.

Haemorrhage Bleeding may occur into the cyst causing a gradual distension and eventually pain and tenderness, as in torsion.

Rupture Rupture may result from torsion or haemorrhage or from an abdominal blow, and if the contents escape into the peritoneal cavity peritonitis may occur.

Infection Infection of a tumour is rare but a genital tract infection following abortion or childbirth may spread to the ovary.

Malignancy Ovarian cysts may undergo malignant changes at any time, but the tendency to do this is greater after the menopause.

Obstruction to labour If the cyst is large it may obstruct the descent of the fetal head into the pelvis during pregnancy and labour, and necessitate a caesarean section combined with the removal of the cyst.

Treatment

The treatment of ovarian cysts depends largely on the age of the patient and whether there are malignant changes or not. Surgery is usually indicated, but when the tumour is malignant this may be combined with radiotherapy or chemotherapy

Malignant ovarian tumours are very difficult to control

therefore there are many different regimes of cytotoxic drugs. Recently, intravenous Cysplatin, administered either alone or combined with other cytotoxic drugs, has given a higher five-year survival to patients.

Operations on the ovary

Ovarian cystectomy Enucleation, or shelling out of the cyst, is the operation of choice in the adolescent and women still in the reproductive phase, because the otherwise healthy ovary can be left. It is an ideal operation for the removal of a dermoid cyst.

Wedge resection of ovary See page 355.

Oophorectomy Removal of an ovary is undertaken in a young woman if the cyst is so large that no recognizable ovarian tissue remains, or in older women for non-malignant tumours. If there is malignant change, a cytotoxic drug such as cyclophosphamide (Endoxana) may be left in the peritoneal cavity at operation, and further doses of cytotoxics may be given intravenously or orally during the postoperative period.

Oophorectomy is usually combined with other operations, such as:

salpingo-oophorectomy—this prevents ectopic pregnancy in the remaining tube (see Chapter 27).

hysterectomy, including Wertheim's hysterectomy (see Chapter 25).

Bilateral oophorectomy The removal of both ovaries has both physiological and physchological effects in causing an artificial menopause, and it is important that the nurse should explain the effects of hormonal changes, if any. (Unilateral oophorectomy has no such effect.) This is discussed on page 217: 'Explanations and Consent'.

The nursing care for all these operations is described in Chapter 19.

CLINICAL USE OF OVARIAN HORMONES

Ovarian hormones are used in gynaecology both palliatively and therapeutically, because of their important actions in the body (see 'General effects of ovarian hormones', Chapter 2). Each condition is described in detail elsewhere in the text, but the indications for use are summarized here.

Oestrogens

Before puberty
   to treat vulvovaginitis (Chapter 22).

During childbearing years
   to inhibit ovulation (Chapter 16)
   to relieve dysmenorrhoea (Chapter 25)
   to restore the oestrogen–progesterone balance, as in metropathia haemorrhagica (Chapter 25)
   to improve cervical mucus (Chapter 15)
   to suppress lactation, but this is becoming rarer now because of the danger of deep vein thrombosis (Chapters 9 and 10)
   to alleviate symptoms such as hot flushes during the menopause (Chapter 17) or after bilateral oophorectomy (page 323).

After the menopause
   to treat senile vaginitis and kraurosis vulvae (Chapter 21).
   Controlled trials using prolonged oestrogen therapy after the menopause have reported excellent results in the prevention of bone fractures in older women.

Progesterone

During childbearing years

to control menorrhagia (Chapter 25)

to relieve symptoms of endometriosis (page 352)

to try to maintain a pregnancy when there is a history of threatened or habitual abortion (Chapter 5)

to reduce fertility, without the side-effects of the combined pill (Chapter 16); or progesterone can be given with oestrogen as oral contraception.

For details of preparations and dosages, a pharmacology textbook should be consulted.

APPENDIX TO CHAPTER 23

Acquired Immune Deficiency Syndrome (AIDS)

AIDS is new to the UK since 1981, but in the USA the incidence has risen rapidly with a mortality rate approaching 100% over two years. AIDS is sexually transmitted and is most often passed between promiscuous homosexuals and to the female partners of bisexual men. However, it also occurs after blood transfusions, in haemophiliacs and in intravenous drug abusers, suggesting that there is an undiscovered blood-borne agent. This has similar implications for nursing management as hepatitis B. AIDS is also spread perinatally to babies of promiscuous intravenous drug abusers.

Patients lack an adequate immune response to fungi, parasites, viruses or bacteria, presenting with Kaposi's sarcoma or opportunist infections.

There is no single diagnostic test, but a lymphocyte count shows lymphopenia (less than 1.5×10^9 per litre).

The management is to treat complications and control infection. Treatment is impossible whilst the underlying cause remains unknown, but spread is controlled in part by reducing homosexual promiscuity and by homosexuals not donating blood.

Herpes Genitalis

Herpes genitalis is an acute viral infection which is being recognized increasingly frequently. Although it appears to be harmless for most patients, there can be serious long-term consequences both for affected adults and for an unborn fetus.

Signs and symptoms The patient first notices a burning discomfort and itching at the affected site: on the vulva, perineum, urethra, periurethral area, introitus, or cervix in women, or on the penis, perpuce or glans in men. This is followed by an erythematous eruption in which several small grouped vesicles appear, which rapidly become eroded forming painful superficial ulcers. Crusting and healing of these normally occurs in 7–14 days, unless there is any secondary infection when they can become deeply ulcerated. There may be some systemic illness.

Diagnosis is confirmed when a swab of material from the ulcers grows herpes simplex virus.

Management Although herpes infections are incurable, viral replication can be inhibited by acyclovir (Zovirax). This controls the disease process, preventing new lesions from forming and halting viral multiplication. Consequently the patient's discomfort is reduced.

The patient should be told that the active lesions transmit the disease by direct sexual contact; and should be warned that the disease may recur, triggered by certain (unknown) stimuli. Recurrences are generally less severe than the primary attack but they can persist for years causing depression and psychosexual problems, with patients often feeling their whole life is wrecked.

Because of a possible link with cervical carcinoma, female patients are advised to have annual smear tests.

Herpes during pregnancy The herpes virus can cross the placenta and enter the fetal circulation, or active lesions can infect a fetus during parturition, causing encephalitis, keratoconjunctivitis or hepatitis, with a mortality of about 60%. Elective caesarian section is therefore often performed when the mother has active genital herpes.

Index